Luci—

My hope is this book will
encourage you. I am an admirer
of you and your wonderful family.

God's best to you. He will
surely help you.
You will recover!

Regg M. Smith

Psalm 84:11

May 30, 2010

# You Can't Fall off the Floor
## (Walking Out of Paralysis)

Ralph M. Smith

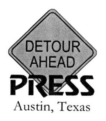

DETOUR
AHEAD
PRESS
Austin, Texas

# In Memoriam

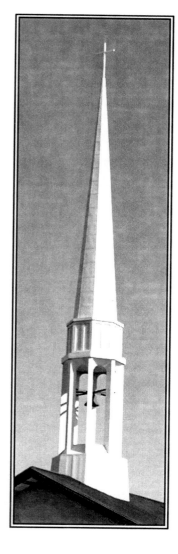

Don Lee Tew
January 3, 1941 – November 20, 2006

*Christian architect and faithful friend*

Don Tew loved his Lord. He loved his family, churches, and children. He dedicated his talents and skills as an architect to designing beautiful buildings for people to worship and for children to learn. He was an encourager.

The Detour Ahead! Foundation would only be a dream without Don's faithful love and support. It's a deep sadness for us that he left this earth for heaven without seeing the fruits from the seeds he sowed.

Steeple designed by

*Don Lee Tew*

Hyde Park Baptist Church
Austin, Texas

iii

# You Can't Fall off the Floor
**By Ralph M. Smith**

© 2008 Ralph M. Smith

Detour Ahead Press
Detour Ahead Foundation Publications
PMB 305
3112 Windsor Road, Suite A
Austin, TX 78703
(512) 328-7685

Library of Congress Control Number:
ISBN: 0-9793542-5-0

First Edition

Senior Editor
Barbara Foley

Editor
Brad Fregger

Book Design & Production
M. Kevin Ford

Cover Design & Production
Original Front Cover Image
M. Kevin Ford

# Dedication

*To my lovely wife Bess, to whom I owe the most, I love you!*

# Foreword

*T*his book chronicles my struggle with Guillian-Barrè Syndrome (pronounced ghee-yan/bahray). It relates how I moved from total paralysis to total independence. I write with the hope this book will give encouragement and hope to someone struggling with paralysis, or any other debilitating illness. Beyond that, I trust the book will encourage family members of the afflicted. My experience is that the families of those who are ill suffer as much, or more, than the patient. They also need reassurance that there is hope beyond paralysis.

I want you to journey with me as I am plunged into paralysis, to cry and laugh with me as we travel through the mysterious illness, Guillian-Barrè Syndrome, and finally to experience my happiness as I walked out of paralysis. Along the way we will have a pity party, laugh at nurses, and struggle with a respirator. We'll even endure the pain of stretching tendons, reviving atrophied muscles, and then learn again how to walk, to swallow food, and to hold a fork. But, in the end, I have faith that the reader of this book will be comforted, cheered, consoled, and assured.

I humbly thank every person mentioned. Without each of you ... I would be in a wheelchair, or worse, paralyzed and bedfast. Each of you kept me alive, gave me hope, and brightened my life.

During the completion of this book, my beloved wife Bess passed on to be with our Lord. This is a terrible loss, one I can hardly stand. However, the years we spent together, and the children that resulted from our union, are the greatest joys of my life.

# Plunged Into Paralysis

*I*t happens so fast!

One moment I am standing by the side of the bed, a second later, I am on the floor. Fortunately, I manage to clutch the bed as I descend. It is a soft landing. Muscles are as weak and limp as wet spaghetti. Straining with all my will, pushing with all my strength, and holding the bed with all my might, I am unable to get up off the floor.

Unfortunately, like an accordion, my legs are folded up under me. I am seated by the side of the bed in an awkward position.

Thinking I must have slipped, I put my hands on the side of the bed to get up. My arms are so weak they cannot push. My fingers will not clutch. My legs are like Jell-O. My brain cannot get my body to respond to the command, "Get on your feet." To my surprise I cannot stand!

Unable to move from the floor, I awaken my wife Bess. She does her best to help me back into the bed, but to no avail.

It must be a stroke! Could it possibly be a heart attack? Whatever the malady is, here I am stuck on the floor. (Looking back, I am glad I did not comprehend my illness, nor realize what was ahead. Not knowing the future is generally good. Knowing would rob one of the happy surprises in tomorrow and keep us worrying about the hard times ahead. One day at a time is enough to handle. The greatest man who ever lived taught: "Sufficient unto the day is the evil thereof.")

My wife phones our family physician, Dr. Richard Helmer. Even though it is 2:30 a.m., Dr. Helmer is kind, helpful, understanding. He is a brilliant internist who specializes in cancer treatment and has been my personal physician for many years. In my opinion, he is the best. Dr. Helmer is mystified regarding my illness. Diagnosing over the phone is at best an educated guess. He suggests that possibly my potassium level has suddenly dropped. Consequently, he prescribes three Slow-K (potassium-chloride) tablets. We are to give them a little time to work. If there is no improvement, he will come to our home.

Later Dr. Helmer tells me, as soon as he put the phone on the receiver he thought, *It is probably Guillian-Barrè Syndrome.*

In about twenty minutes I feel better. With the help of Bess, I crawl into bed and go back to sleep. I can raise

2

my arms over my head but cannot turn over, and I am still unable to stand. Something within my body is not functioning properly. We are anticipating it is not serious. My being able to get back into bed is to us a good sign. Perhaps sleep will restore my strength.

At 5:30 a.m. I awaken. My head is hurting. My bladder is about to explode. I have always had a small bladder. Years ago traveling in Israel I learned never to pass a public restroom. It may be a long time before the bus stops again. Nothing is so underrated as a good trip to the toilet!

Cautiously, I again attempt to walk. Clutching the bed I once more slip helplessly to the floor. Bess brings me a jar, and I quickly fill it with urine. Greatly relieved, a second time I attempt to crawl into bed. My arms are so weak I cannot lift myself. My legs are inoperative. Obviously, I am not getting any better. Once again, I am lying on the floor beside my bed. I cannot get up and Bess is unable to get me back into the bed.

I have become much weaker. Bess again phones Dr. Helmer describing my condition. Realizing it is more serious than first assumed, he tells her to call the Emergency Medical System (EMS) for an ambulance to take me to Seton Hospital; he will meet us in the emergency room.

In a very short time EMS is at our front door. Three paramedics enter our bedroom and go through the normal routine; checking pulse, blood pressure, eyes, throat, etc. These people are most efficient. Soon they are convinced I have not suffered a heart attack...comforting! Stroke is still a real option ... depressing!

We are perplexed as to my malady. Soon the guessing game will end. Later I learn that a stroke or heart attack would have been a welcome relief, compared to the world of pain, uncertainty, and frustration I am about to enter.

Life is short and fickle. It is best not to take any one event too seriously. The next ten or twenty minutes are humorous. I am thinking, *No heart attack ... no stroke ... everything will soon be fine ... after all I have hardly ever been sick. I'm sure it's a virus ... a shot of penicillin and I will be up and running.*

It is difficult for me to remember many days when I was sick. As a child I had measles three or four days. Mumps was my longest illness. It was a steamy-hot Arkansas summer and I had to stay in bed four or five days. Beyond those childhood illnesses, I was the picture of health. I never broke a bone, except for a fractured jaw playing high school football. The doctor found it unnecessary to wire my jaws shut. I could not, however, chew food for six weeks. I took nourishment through a straw. The broken jaw became an excuse to drink chocolate milkshakes, which did not seem bad to a sixteen-year-old. That summarizes my childhood and youth illnesses.

Good health is in my genes, a gift of God. Seldom did I do much to encourage my body to be healthy. When you have good health, you tend to take it for granted. I did. I believed my excellent state of health would last forever. Unfortunately, on that day I learned that I, too, am a frail, weak, mortal human. I discovered I could be stricken suddenly and my world could take on a new dimension.

I am flat on my back, on the floor, cradled between the bed and wall. The paramedics are having a discussion about how they can wedge me out, and lift me up to the gurney. This is no small challenge. I weigh well over two-hundred pounds. They are working in a confined area. Due to my weakness, I am of no assistance. Since I can do nothing to help, I listen to their conversation with keen interest.

Here are two men and a woman with three different opinions. Apparently, they are frustrated. Probably they have already worked all night. I am their last patient for this shift. How can they wedge me out? Though paralyzed and hurting, I am amused. After fifteen minutes, the paramedics manage to shuffle me around to a position where they can lift me onto the gurney.

This being accomplished, they wheel me out of the house and into the ambulance. Riding in an ambulance on a flat plastic board is hard on the spine. Every turn in the road is an adventure. Bumps register from the top of the head, down the spine, and into the heels of the feet. It is an eight, or nine, on the Richter Scale. This is the longest short ride I have ever taken!

Strangest of all is the feeling of shame I am experiencing. I am ashamed I am having to be transported in an emergency vehicle to the hospital. My wish is that I see no one who knows me. It is my first realization that when illness strikes, particularly paralysis, there is a sense of shame. (After my illness for many months, psychologically, I will feel inferior. Being not as strong as I once was allows this inferiority complex to creep into my mind. Have you ever observed that many crippled and paralyzed people habitually look down?)

By the time the ambulance arrives at Seton Hospital I am unable to move any of my extremities. I am paralyzed from my neck to the soles of my feet. My feelings are of helplessness, frustration, and shame. I can cope with the helplessness and frustration. What is puzzling me is this nagging feeling of shame. Really, there should be no shame when a person is sick. Nevertheless, my overriding feeling is one of abasement.

After being rolled into the hospital emergency ward, I am parked in a small area cordoned off by white draw curtains. Dr. Helmer has already arrived and examines me. He informs Bess that he has called Dr. Michael Douglas, a prominent neurologist in Austin. Within a brief time Dr. Douglas arrives and introduces himself. After scanning my chart he asks a number of questions. His diagnosis is that I have Guillain-Barrè Syndrome (GBS). Neither Bess nor I have ever heard of this strange-sounding illness. Dr. Douglas indicates his diagnosis could be confirmed, or ruled out, by a spinal tap. The presence of protein in the spinal column indicates GBS.

My next stop is the imaging room. Having never had a spinal tap, I do not know what to expect. When I was a child I remember our family physician relating how one doctor permanently paralyzed a patient doing a spinal tap. Even though that was fifty or more years ago, and there has been colossal medical progress, I am apprehensive. The specter of fear has entered my mind.

Apparently, the young physician who is to perform the spinal tap senses my apprehension. He suggests I watch the TV monitor. He is reassuring. Sensing I am still nervous, he boasts he is the best in the business. This helps. I like people who believe in themselves. There is nothing wrong with self-confidence. Nevertheless, I am still uneasy.

A long hypodermic needle is about to be inserted into my spine. Spinal fluid will be extracted to determine if there is protein in my spinal column. Watching the monitor is comforting. However, I avoid hypodermic needles like the plague. For me, one-hundred pills swallowed five at a time is preferable to one shot. Little do I know that for the next six months my body will become a pincushion for hypodermic needles.

No one can convince me that nurses do not enjoy giving injections. They seem to have a sadistic streak. Beyond that they have little sense of *your* pain. Before injecting a needle they usually say, "This won't hurt." What they really mean is, it won't hurt *them*.

Skillfully the young physician inserts the needle into my spine. The procedure, I had imagined torturous and life-threatening, is nearly painless. There is protein! The spinal tap confirms I have GBS.

What is Guillain-Barrè Syndrome? Is it serious? Will I recover? How long will recovery take? Is it contagious? I have a barrage of questions, but this is neither the time nor the place to ask them. I am about to be wheeled into a Neurological Critical Care Unit (NCC).

Later I read articles that give an insight into the definition the medical profession gives Guillain-Barrè Syndrome. *Syndrome* is the term used to describe the illness, rather than disease. This reflects the recognition of the illness by the collection of symptoms told to the doctor by the patient, and signs observed by the physician upon examining the patient that typify the disorder. It is a rare and mysterious illness that affects the peripheral nerves of the body. Weakness is its main characteristic. Paralysis and abnormal sensations often follow. At the moment I am experiencing every GBS symptom … and more!

GBS was first diagnosed in 1916 by three French physicians: George Guillain, Jean Barrè, and Andre Stohl. The way had been opened by Quinke in 1891. He demonstrated spinal fluid can be removed by inserting a needle into the lower back.

When a spinal tap reveals the characteristic abnormality of increased fluid proteins, with normal cell count, GBS is identified. It can affect nerves not only to the limbs and breathing muscles, but also those to the throat, heart, urinary bladder, and eyes. Doctors have any number of ways to describe GBS. They may say it is "acute idiopathic polyneuritis." Translated this means: a rapid onset of unknown cause resulting in irritation or inflammation of many nerves.

Nerves that extend from the spinal cord outward are called peripheral nerves. Some of these nerves are covered, such as electric wires are in our home, by insulation. This sheath insulation covering the nerves is called myelin. In GBS, the myelin is damaged. This damage slows down, or short-circuits, the ability of the nerves to conduct a signal normally. The slowed signal causes the patient to experience weakness. If conduction is too slow, or blocked, the patient may become paralyzed.

That is my condition. I am *totally* paralyzed. Insulation around my nerves has been severely damaged. I can open and close my eyes, barely twitch a finger, and slightly move a hand. This is the extent of my movement.

Since I slipped onto the floor early this morning, I have progressively become weaker. The myelin sheath apparently is gone from my nerves. I silently think, *Ralph, remember, a live wire usually burns the insulation off.* ...

GBS cannot be predicted. It came into my life at age sixty-four. It can occur at any age and in both sexes. It is sporadic. It varies greatly in severity. Some mild cases may never be brought to the doctor's attention. Unfortunately, mine is an extremely severe case. Already it has me in complete paralysis. As many as five percent of those with this illness die; being sixty-four years of age is not in my favor.

The cause of GBS is not known at this time. There was an outbreak of GBS when President Gerald Ford urged Americans to take the swine-flu vaccine. My GBS followed shortly after I took a flu vaccine. It is my belief this vaccine triggered or caused my GBS. There appears to be a correlation between the two.

GBS is a disorder of the nervous system. When we decide to perform some activity, such as walking, the brain sends an electric signal down the nerve path in the spinal cord. This signal, in turn, is conducted out of the spinal cord by nerves that go to the muscles. The nerves that extend from the spinal cord outwards are peripheral nerves. These are the nerves that are impaired by GBS. This damage slows down or short-circuits the ability of the nerve to conduct a signal normally. With the slowed signal I am weakened, and finally paralyzed.

Not only are the nerves to and from my limbs affected, but nerves from the spinal column to the chest muscles are being attacked. These muscles affect respiration. Later other parts of my autonomic system will be affected, particularly kidneys.

One good thing is that in GBS the brain and spinal cord do not appear to be affected. Thus my brain function remains normal, as well as short nerves coming out of my brain to my ears and nose. I can think, hear, and smell normally. For several months opening and closing my eyes will be the *one* exercise I can do efficiently.

The *Fort Worth Star Telegram* carried an article on my illness. Accurately, the writer stated I am "a mind imprisoned in a body." GBS, fortunately, does not at-

11

tack the brain function. With all the other complications I am having, I remain extremely grateful my mind is unaffected.

I recall one of my wife's favorite stories.

A man is ill. The doctor diagnoses his illness, then tells him he will need a brain transplant. The patient is unaware this is possible. The physician says it is, but he will have to make a choice. He can get a man's brain transplanted for $95,000, or a woman's brain for $20,000. The patient asks, "Why is the man's brain so much more expensive?"

The surgeon responds, "The man's brain has never been used."

In the coming weeks my brain will be stretched and exercised to its limit. Helpless and paralyzed, I am forced to utilize all my brain power to stay alert, avoid depression, keep a positive attitude, and refrain from asking unanswerable questions. The mind is like a muscle and can atrophy, shrivel, decay. "Use it or lose it" applies to mind and muscle alike. In the ensuing months my greatest battle will be between my ears, in my brain, because there I will determine whether I remain a helpless cripple, or return to being a robust man.

This paralysis, that has me flat on my back and helpless, came like a bolt of lighting out of the sky. There were no warning signs of this impending illness ... or were there forewarnings?

12

There were two brothers who were totally dedicated to their manufacturing business. Thus they never married. Rich and successful, neither would even take time for a vacation. One brother said, "You need a vacation. Here is a first-class, round-trip ticket to Paris. I reserved a suite for you in a five-star hotel. You leave this weekend. The trip is my gift to you. Have a great holiday!"

His shocked bachelor brother responds, "I can't go."

"Why not?"

"Who will take care of my cat?"

His brother replies, "I will care for your cat. Go!"

Reluctantly, the brother departs for Paris. For a week he has a wonderful time, but then he begins to worry about his cat. He phones his brother asking, "How is my cat?"

"Your cat died."

The next day is miserable. All he can do is mourn over his dead cat. Again he phones his brother saying, "You were cruel telling me my cat died."

"What should I have done?"

"Well, you should have prepared me for her death. When I phoned, you could have said, 'The cat is on the roof.' The next day when I phoned, you could have told me the cat fell off the roof and is at the veterinarian clinic. Then the next day when I called, you could have said, 'The veterinarian did everything possible, but your cat died.' I would have been prepared."

"I am sorry. ..."

Then the vacationing brother asks, "How is mother?"

"Mother is on the roof. ..."

A warning is not always helpful. On reflection, there were harbingers about a coming illness.

Many weeks before I was stricken, a red scab appeared on the back of my left hand, where my thumb and first finger join. The scab would not go away. At my wife's insistence I made an appointment with our dermatologist, Dr. William Green.

Dr. Green examined my hand and had several ideas as to what the red scab was. He was convinced the only way to be certain was by collecting a small sample for biopsies. He has never led me wrong, so I agreed to have it analyzed. On my return visit a week later, Dr. Green stated the biopsy revealed I had Sweet's Syndrome. He went on to say this indicated a latent problem. He named a number of possibilities and suggested I have a complete physical examination. His final statement was, "Ralph, you have a potential illness. We just do not know what it is."

Following Dr. Green's suggestion, I was given a complete physical examination. No abnormalities were discovered. In the ensuing weeks I found my strength was diminishing. By the end of the day, I was exhausted. It seemed difficult to walk up stairs. I found myself taking short naps in the afternoon, something I have never done before. Twice I thought I had a viral infection, or the flu. I was not well, but I was not sick enough to be in bed.

14

When GBS is finally diagnosed Dr. Douglas says, "Ralph, had we known it was coming, we could not have prevented it." That is both comforting and shocking. GBS is an enigmatic malady.

The latest research indicates, regardless of the triggering event, the nerves of the Guillian-Barrè patient are attacked by the body's own defense system against disease, antibodies, and white blood cells. The result is that the myelin sheath covering the nerves of the patient is damaged, or eaten away.

The illness is an enigma, even to the best physicians. Faced with a mysterious situation, we all have different coping mechanisms. It has never helped me to cope by blaming myself, or someone else. I am old enough, and hopefully mature enough, to not ask, *"Why?"* It is counterproductive to become angry with God.

Faced with a tragic circumstance, we are inclined to ask, "Why did this happen to me?" Often there is only capricious speculation. If we knew the answer, the next question we would ask is another, "Why?" The right question is not, "Why?" but, *"What* can I do now? *Where* do I go for help? *How* do I get well? *When* will I recover?"

Not once have I ever asked God, my doctors, or myself, "Why did this happen to me?" That will forever remain the unanswered question of life. My thought pattern is quite simple:

> *Things are not as bad as they seem.*
> *Things could be worse.*
> *Things will get better.*

It works for me! Flat on my back, paralyzed by a mysterious illness, I say to myself, *Ralph, it's okay; one day you are going to walk out of this paralysis.*

# A Mind Imprisoned in a Body

$\mathcal{E}$ ven though I know next to nothing about GBS, it is obvious I am getting progressively weaker; the GBS is attacking my lungs and breathing has become more difficult. I have now been in the hospital only six hours and I am already on a mouth respirator. A tube is placed in my mouth that extends into my throat. The opening is securely taped to my cheeks and is attached to a machine that pumps air into my lungs.

I must be a slow learner. It took me a few hours to realize: *I am on a life-support system. The tracheal tube is keeping me alive! Without it I am unable to breathe.*

The next four or five days are a blur. On a scale of one to ten, my pain level is eleven. I hurt from the top of my bald head to the tip of my big toe. Being understanding and compassionate, my doctors keep me heavily sedated. It is hard to stay awake. The whole experience is like a bad dream, a nightmare. I am in a fog.

Since I am on a respirator, it has become necessary to feed me without food going through my mouth. For a brief time I am fed intravenously (IV). A few days later a nasoenteral tube is inserted. Patients who need short-term internal nutritional support usually have either a nasogastric (NG) tube, which is inserted through the nose and into the stomach, or a nasointestinal (NI) tube, which extends into the distal duodenum or proximal jejunum. Since my food did not need to bypass the stomach, the natural and preferred feeding site, a nasogastric tube is inserted.

In layman's terms, the doctor has inserted a tube through my nose into my stomach. Three or more times daily the attending nurses pour Ensure into the tube. This has become my nutrition. It is invariably vanilla. I can't talk, so I cannot request chocolate or strawberry. Since it doesn't enter my mouth, I realize I cannot taste it anyway. Flavor matters little when feeding is through a nose tube that extends into the stomach. Still, I prefer chocolate, but I am unable to make my request known.

Beyond the tracheal tube and nasal feeding tube, I am wired. An oxymeter is attached to my left index finger. It measures the oxygen content in my blood. Additionally, I am placed on a heart monitor. Pods are glued to my chest, checking the vital functions of my heart. Flat on my back from the corner of my left eye, I can see a nurse checking the heart monitor, blood pressure, pulse, etc. She, or one of her associates, is there twenty-four hours a day, and appears always busy.

18

Since I am unable to get out of bed, a catheter is inserted to drain urination. I am more helpless than a newborn baby. A baby is able to move its arms and legs. I can do neither; consequently, the nurses care for me like a baby. I am sixty-four years of age and in diapers. Sick, dependent, helpless, and frustrated best describe my state of being.

Endlessly, nurses are sticking needles in me. They are giving blood, taking blood, or injecting medicine. I feel like a pincushion. "Dracula" comes regularly every morning to draw blood. It appears to me the nurses stick needles in me just to stay in practice. I am a good candidate. I can't talk, so I can't complain. That is good because I might say things to the nurses unbecoming to a southern gentleman. My greatest medical dread is being pricked with a hypodermic needle. This phobia is being severely tested.

My treatment consists of Plasma Pharisees. In this procedure the blood is changed out or cleansed to rid it of bad antibodies. GBS is a puzzling illness. Consequently, a "sure cure" has not been discovered. Treatment is day-by-day, depending on the condition of the patient. Doctors are exact in describing their profession—they refer to it as the *practice* of medicine. I am giving them a stellar opportunity to "practice."

The mouth tracheal tube is agitating my raw sore throat. The sensation is that there is hot sand in my windpipe. There is a gremlin rubbing the sand against my throat. I want to spit but can't.

Additionally, I cannot talk. Can you imagine how frustrating it is to a preacher not to be able to talk? Talking is my business. Right now, I am out of business. My life is like a sign I once saw on an elevator that read: NOT WORKING TODAY. That describes me—not working today, or the next, or the next.

Everything in NCC frustrates me. I definitely do not like being here! My whole body tingles and aches. At the same time it feels numb. When anyone touches me anywhere, I want to scream. Only the mouth tracheal tube stifles my outcry. I am still in a fog. I feel terrible. Someone is always waking me when I want to sleep, and telling me to sleep when I want to be awake.

Time moves slowly in NCC. There is no clock on the wall. Calendars would be more appropriate. Medicine flows one drop at a time from the IV bottle. Days and nights are jumbled. I cannot tell AM from PM unless someone informs me. I never know which day of the week it is. Time is measured by family's and doctor's visits. I know it is early morning when "Dracula" comes to draw blood, or the x-ray technicians lift me to place an x-ray plate under my stiff, sore back.

20

With the tracheal tube in my throat, I cannot even look forward to meal time and the pleasant sensation of chewing food. I am unable to do anything. Doing nothing is very tiring. You can never stop and take a rest.

Being unable to do anything physically, my mind is active. My first thought, other than frustration, is: *Now is my great opportunity to develop patience.* All my life it has been in short supply. Patience is a beautiful virtue I do not possess. The Bible teaches: "... tribulation brings patience." This makes me reluctant to pray for patience.

I am like the man who cut six holes in the bottom of his kitchen door. A visitor asks him, "Why six holes in the door?"

"The six holes are there because I have six cats. The holes allow them to come and go."

The visitor says, "You only need one hole. All the cats can come and go through the same opening."

The cat lover responds, "When I say scat, I mean scat!"

That describes my impatience. I have always thought one of the world's greatest inventions is *instant* coffee. I am frustrated when I miss one turn of a revolving door. My impatience and agitation with NCC is creating anxiety. My wife Bess tells me the doctors are more concerned about my anxiety than the GBS. Years ago I read that stress is a leading cause of illness. It can cause numerous afflictions including: headaches, heart attacks, ulcers, etc. Anxiety is working on me and not helping my situation.

I have been in the hospital only three days and my blood pressure is nearing 200. Normally my blood pressure is low. Mentally I am not handling this illness well. I am too sick to care. Anxiety is gripping my mind. I think, *I will have to get better to die.* My positive thinking has gone negative. Fighting depression, I am losing.

A downcast man talks with his friend about being depressed. He says, "I think it is a bad day."
> The friend responds, "Be positive."
> "OK, I am positive it is a bad day!"

Treatment in NCC is wearing me out. I cannot move. I sleep all day. My progress is in reverse. It is a vicious cycle. My frustration leads to anxiety. The anxiety results in further frustration. I am in a revolving door of frustration-anxiety-frustration. Stress is a crippling illness. It is in the process of destroying me.

My sixth day in the hospital, I catch pneumonia. Mine is not just any old strain of pneumonia. The germ I have is very rare, and consequently, resistant to most drugs. It is resisting whatever my doctor first prescribed. Vancomycin is administered but the afternoon x-rays are worse than those in the morning. Progress is in reverse.

Life is challenging with a tracheal tube in my mouth and pneumonia slowly drowning my lungs.

I reason that this is one more step in my dying process.

Reading the comic strip, "The Wizard of Id," I found the very short king conferring with a clairvoyant. Gazing into her crystal ball she says to the king, "I see you in a funeral procession."

The king inquires, "At the front or rear?"

Given the choice right now, I would elect to lead the funeral procession, carried by six good friends. For the first time in my life I am having a death wish. Neither my doctors nor my family know I am hoping I will die. Though I have never agreed with what the man does, I catch myself thinking, *Where is Dr. Kevorkian when you need him?*

That is sick thinking. When an individual entertains a death wish, that person is thinking illogically. I have slipped, no plunged, into deep melancholia. My depression is in the depths. My mind is confused.

Treatment for GBS is halted. I am too weak to have Plasma Pharisees, where the blood is changed out to rid it of bad antibodies. The doctors continue to be more concerned about my anxiety than the syndrome. I am thinking, *Tomorrow will be a brighter day*...and then it rains.

One week after my being admitted to the hospital, Dr. Douglas decides to move the tracheal tube to my throat, if my pneumonia is better. During the night my breathing becomes so labored that an emergency tracheotomy is performed. Waiting until morning might prove to be fatal. My physical condition is weaker with every fleeting hour.

My wife signs the papers for the tracheotomy. Though fearful, I am relieved. With things as they are, I will have that death wish granted. Early in the evening Dr. Richard Denton is summoned to install the tracheotomy tube in my throat. In about one hour he successfully completes the procedure. The surgical procedure is performed in my NCC room. I am so sick, I do not remember anything about it. I am extremely happy when it is over. The tracheal tube that had been in my mouth brought more discomfort than the tracheotomy tube now in my throat.

Even after having my throat slit, I sleep soundly. Later I tell a number of people, "If you are going to have your throat slit, call Dr. Denton. He is the best!" I wish I could still say, "Call Dr. Denton." Unfortunately, Dr. Denton has since been taken home to Heaven. He was one great, dedicated physician. Always gentle, kind, and compassionate, he personified what a doctor should be. Heaven is richer and Earth poorer for his death.

24

Upon waking I rediscover that the tracheal tube is no longer in my mouth. That is good. But, now a tracheotomy tube is in my throat. That is bad. This reminds me of a story told by Dr. Pat Neff, former Governor of Texas and former President of Baylor University.

A forty-year-old bachelor finally got married. He went home to announce his marriage to his aged father, "Dad, I finally got married."
"Son, that is good!"
"Yes, but my wife is ugly."
"Son, that is bad."
"But my wife is extremely rich."
"That is good!"
"But Dad, she is very stingy."
"Son, that is bad!"
"Yes, but she built us a million-dollar house."
"That is good!"
"But the house burned down."
"Son, that is bad!"
"Yes, but she was in it!"
And the dad did not know what to say.

Eight days have now elapsed since I was brought to NCC. I am not sleeping well at night. Rest is essential to my recovery. Shakespeare wisely penned: "Sleep knits up the raveled sleeve of care ... ."

The realization is sinking into my mind that this could take some time. Easter is coming and I grasp I will not be able to lead our church in worship. Like it or not, I am going to have to develop patience.

In order to prevent foot drop, the nurses put black high-top tennis shoes on me. I am not sure they are really shoes, but they resemble shoes. I have never preferred tennis shoes. In fact, I never wear high-top shoes. Who wears black tennis shoes? These are not my style and this ups my frustration level. Have you ever tried to sleep with your shoes on? My pulse shoots up to 123, extremely high for me.

This evening Bess and my daughter Diane visit. How thrilled I am when the family is allowed to visit. They tell me I appear upset and agitated. I cannot move. With the trachea, I cannot talk. Last night I had surgery. I have just begun to understand I can't lead the Easter worship service. A week in NCC can seem like a lifetime. Apparently I am distraught. By 9:00 p.m. Bess and Diane can no longer bear seeing my distress. They have to leave.

Good riddance! I am so sick, I don't care. My prevailing thought is, *Can't they realize I am dying? All of this is pointless ... and they observe I am upset ... what other brilliant observations have they made?*

The next day is filled with highs and lows. I am like an elevator operator whose work has its ups and downs.

26

I will take pleasure from the mountain top of hope, and then slide into the valley of discouragement. Dr. Douglas tells my wife I am right on track neurologically, but my lungs are not in very good shape. He states I will recover, if I do not develop serious complications.

GBS has taken possession of another small part of my anatomy. The left side of my face is now paralyzed. The doctor, however, thinks he saw movement on the right side of my body. He is mistaken.

The medical team decides to hold off on Plasma Pharisees. Instead they start IVGG. This treatment consists of giving massive doses of gamma globulin. I do not know why this decision is made. On second thought, I do not understand anything being done, which bothers me. In my case, however, ignorance is bliss. Not knowing is bad, and knowing what is ahead would be worse!

My blood pressure is down but my pulse is abnormally high. The morning x-ray indicates my chest is worse than the day before. The pneumonia is rugged. It is not responding to the Vancomycin. Dr. Douglas confirms that the pulmonary doctors will determine what additional treatment to give, if any. I think, *He believes I am going to die, though wisely he indicates to Bess I will improve. Truth is, I, too, believe I will die.*

The IVGG is possibly the best and last medication available to control GBS. It, however, doesn't seem to help. My breathing is laborious, even with the respirator.

At this very low point, my family tells me I am belligerent. I want to say to them, "I can please one person per day. Today is not your day. Tomorrow isn't looking good either."

My thought is, *How can they know how I feel? I can't speak a word. I am ... paralyzed, helpless.* On reflection I realize they are accurate in their assessment of my mood. I am angry with the family, doctors, nurses, and hospital staff. I had told my wife *never* to put me on life support machines. Specifically, I am angry with my wife, whom I love more than life. No one could have a better mate. As far as I am concerned, my wife is perfect. That is the very reason I am irate! Knowing how much my wife loves me, how can she allow the doctors to artificially sustain my life?

My breathing is sustained by a respirator. They are feeding me through a tube inserted in my nose going into my stomach. My urination is through a catheter, which continually irritates me. I am wearing diapers, because I can neither use a bed pan, nor go to the commode. A pulse oxymeter is on my finger measuring oxygen content in the blood stream. On my feet are ugly black shoes intended to prevent drop foot. My body is rigid in paralysis.

I cannot twitch a finger, move a foot, turn my head, shift from side to side, or talk. I am in severe physical pain. A nurse is camped outside my room twenty-four hours a day, watching monitors keeping me alive.

*Yes, I feel lousy. I sense I am dying.*

I am drowning in a well, in a canyon of depression, at the bottom of the ocean. I am in the deep pit of despair. My overriding thought is, *Why don't they let me die?* Death would be a welcome relief from what I am experiencing. Any time a nurse touches me, I want to scream. Have you ever gone to a dentist and he hit a raw nerve with his drill? This is the feeling I am experiencing all over my body. The insulation of my peripheral nerves has been eaten away. Those exposed nerves are highly sensitive.

Like the reporter for the *Fort Worth Star Telegram* wrote, I am a mind imprisoned in a body. My good friend, Ed Perry, says Congress should pass a law so that an individual can declare himself to be a horse. When a horse is sick and suffering, the veterinarian gives the animal an injection and puts it out of its pain. At this moment, I would like to declare myself a horse. I am miserably in pain.

X-rays reveal I have more fluid on my lungs. The pneumonia is threatening to grant my wish for death. Dr. Weingarten comes to aid my labored breathing. The kind doctor removes the tracheotomy tube attached to my throat. He takes a long rubber tube and inserts it into the trachea throat hole, slipping it into my lung. Suction is applied and water is drained from one lung, then the other. During the procedure I cannot breathe. This will become a routine procedure happening often for the remainder of my stay in NCC.

The first time Dr. Weingarten suctions my lungs, I mentally flee to "Panic Palace." I cognize, *I am going to drown!* It is the most frightening thing I have ever experienced. Unfortunately, the nurses will now do this procedure every few hours. They routinely suction water and mucus from my lungs night and day. I will not have more than two to three hours of continuous sleep for the next half year.

This suctioning of my lungs is horrible! It normally lasts only twenty to forty seconds. During that time I can't breathe. These few seconds seem eternal in duration. It is physical maltreatment and mental agony. The sensation is one of drowning.

Along with the hardships of life, there is always good occurring. The hospital brings me an Effica Bed. It is the Cadillac, Lexus, and Rolls Royce of hospital beds. It rotates my body. It moves in waves to rest the body. It is fully adjustable, allowing me to sit up straight, or elevate any part of my body. Additionally, it weighs me. It is so effective, that after being in the hospital six months, I will not have a single bed sore. That is a minor miracle.

30

# The Daily Routine

*M*ore than anything else the daily routine of NCC is grinding me down and wearing me out. Every morning promptly at 5:30, two x-ray technicians awaken me, if I am still asleep. They crank up my bed to get me in a partial sitting position. They lift my shoulders and place a half-inch thick plate under my back. Lifting me and sliding the plate under my back is difficult for them and painful for me. The x-ray plate seems to bore into my shoulder and back. Since I have pneumonia with fluid building in my lungs, this is an essential procedure. Doctors need to be aware of the fluid increasing or decreasing in my lungs.

The multitude of x-rays taken should either: (1) kill all potential cancer cells in my lungs or (2) someday cause me to have cancer. The jury is out on which is accomplished with the daily x-rays.

Following the x-rays, several routines take place that get me off to a bad start for the day. The lab technician draws blood from my arm. As you now know, drawing blood heads the list of my dislikes. Reluctantly, I admit I have nearly fainted in my doctor's office when blood was drawn. It is reported a mouse can scare an elephant. A hypodermic needle frightens me.

After this, the nurse cleans my tracheotomy tube. During this process I am not breathing well, if at all. The nurse then pours water into my nose-feeding tube to clean it. Following the cleansing, I am fed Ensure through the tube. It remains consistently vanilla.

By the time this ends, I am exhausted but unable to rest. An LVN drains the bag holding my urine and checks the catheter. Then she and another nurse change my diaper and bathe me. These procedures usually involve three nurses. They must turn me on my side and lift me. My myelin sheath has been eaten away by the GBS, so the nerves are exposed. A touch hurts, so turning and bathing me is akin to being in a medieval torture chamber. Tears fill my eyes and I try to remember, "....pain endures but for a moment."

Now I am x-rayed, injected, suctioned, diapered, fed, bathed, and dressed in a hospital gown (with southern exposure). It's probably not yet 8:00 a.m. but I am exhausted, drained of strength and energy. I do not know what day it is. I have lost all track of time, day, and date.

My doctors come by to check on me. There are several. Each doctor spends a few minutes reading charts outside my room. Some enter my room, but most simply move on to the next patient. When a doctor does enter the room he asks, "How are you doing?"

Silence is the answer.

Since I can't talk with the tracheotomy tube in my throat, the question is rhetorical. I have always wondered why a dentist asks his patient a question when he has both hands and a drill in the patient's mouth.

Daily my neurologist, Dr. Douglas, visits. He pulls up the sheet and asks, "Can you move your toes?" Again, I cannot talk. He tells me to shrug my shoulders. I cannot do that either. He now departs without covering my exposed body with the sheet he removed.

My body is paralyzed, but my mind is overactive. The thought pattern is up and down. My first thought is, *Why do the doctors allow me to live paralyzed on a life-support system?* My second thought is, *My family knows I do not want to be just a vegetable. I am going to either die or end up bedfast and paralyzed. Why do they not insist on pulling the plug?*

Yet, my friends have convinced me I am going to live. Attempting to peer into my future, I wonder, *Would not death be a better alternative?*

My mind is locked on permanently being incapacitated, should I survive the GBS. My doctors, friends, and family are cautiously optimistic I will eventually get well. The question haunting my mind is, *What do they mean when they say I will get well?*

Since I can do nothing physically except be alive, I am reflecting, reasoning, and pondering what my future will become. If I do manage to survive, I will most likely be disabled. At best, I will survive my illness with a severe handicap. Life does not hold a very promising future.

Of even greater concern to me is my wife. She is precious. All her adult life she has worked and sacrificed for me, our children, and the church. The "love of my life" does not deserve to be saddled with a helpless quadriplegic.

Moreover, what kind of a physical and financial burden will I be to our three children and their families? Dealing with me in old age is one issue. Helping a quadriplegic is a far greater responsibility.

All of these negative and pessimistic thoughts are turning in my brain.

Struggling to breathe and fighting for life, this undetected greater conflict is taking place. It occupies center stage in my mind. How can I cope with the impending probability that I may not die, but instead get well? How do I handle the ominous possibility of lifelong severe physical limitations? It now appears, if I live, I will be bedfast, sustained by an oxygen tube the remainder of my life. I may get well ... with severe handicaps!

There is little optimism regarding my future physical condition. How can I maintain an optimistic outlook? I decide to reflect on history. This becomes the key to facing my potential dark and enigmatic future.

Why did I choose to major in history during college? Perhaps so I could work through the prospect of future disability. History can be a great teacher. While in intensive care struggling to breathe and fighting for life, I recognize that unless a person is a rare exception, he or she is handicapped in some way. Those boring college history classes will become one means of deliverance from doubt regarding my future.

The biographies of famous successful men and women confirm many, if not most, were handicapped. Beethoven, while stone deaf, wrote classical music. Milton wrote poetry, though blind. Modern medicine rests on the work of Pasteur. He had a paralytic stroke at the age of forty-six.

The list is endless of histories famous who struggled with a handicap. Julius Caesar had epilepsy. Charles Darwin was an invalid. Lord Nelson had only one eye. Charles Steinmetz was a hunchback. Robert Lewis Stevenson had tuberculosis. President Franklin Delano Roosevelt had polio (some now believe he had GBS) and ran the United States government from a wheelchair during the dark days of World War II. Yet all of them overcame disadvantage and reached the fulfillment of their dreams. Their handicaps became stepping stones to achievement.

Biographies in the Bible parallel history. Joseph spent nearly eighteen years in an Egyptian prison. Later he became prime minister of that nation. Job lost wealth, health, and seven children in tragedy. He is the model on how to suffer successfully. Even the Apostle Paul had a thorn in the flesh. This was a limitation he could not evade, prayed to escape, but he had to settle down and live with it somehow or another. He prayed earnestly for its removal. It stayed. He discovered God's grace was sufficient, writing thirteen books in the Bible and planting churches throughout Asia Minor and Europe.

There are millions of people who are deaf or hard of hearing. Many more than that need glasses or contact lenses. Millions are crippled. Myriads have cancer, diabetes, heart ailments, ulcers, or some other nagging illness. Add to that list those who are crippled by divorce, being out of work, mental illness, poverty, or depression. Hardship is the rule, not the exception.

The fastest-growing segment of our population is the eighty-plus group. Hundreds of thousands, because of old age, are unable to be as active as they desire. I have not yet known a man or woman, who on intimate acquaintance, did not turn out to be dealing with some handicap.

Among the few things that are true of all of us is the fact that each of us has a handicap. It is a crucial moment of realization in my life. Open-eyed, I face my limitation, and admit I possibly will be disabled for the rest of my life.

Apparently, I have joined the multitudes with disability. The question is, "Will I be a coward or a hero? Will I conquer my handicap or will my impediment defeat me?" The challenge before me poses a query regarding my internal makeup. Often I have reminded myself: *Quitters never win, and winners never quit.*

At issue is whether I believe the adage, or merely quote it.

From this point on there will be ups and downs, but in my mind the outcome will never be uncertain. My dream and drive will be to get as well as I possibly can. If there remains some limitation, I will rise above it, and live with it joyfully.

I have not come to this decision quickly. It has taken three months of mental struggle, sometimes praying for death, before I decide I want to live. Additionally, my decision does not infer I will not be discouraged, devastated, and depressed in the future. If anyone ever had a death wish, I am that person. On reflection, my death wish was a mistake. But it did lead me to some deeper convictions.

*I have zero control over anything.* This deepens my faith in God. Truth is, He is ultimately in control of everything. Even when well, and I thought I had control of my life, I didn't. God kept the universe in balance to make Earth habitable. He gave me one lung full of air at a time and made my heart palpitate to sustain my life. I am so weak that a tiny organism can invade my body and put me flat on my back. Why did I ever believe I was in control?

Often I cannot control what happens in life. All I can control is my reaction to it. Struggling in NCC my perspective is going up and down like a yo-yo. I want to live. Then becoming depressed, I pray to die. All of my strength, willpower, and the medical help administered are insufficient. I need strength from God. I will be defeated by what is around me, if I am not strengthened by that which is above me.

Had I a choice, I would not choose to be so desperately sick, helpless, and paralyzed. *Few people get their first choice.* To take second best and make something of it—is success.

The great violinist, Ole Bull, was giving a concert in Paris. His "A" string snapped in the midst of the concert. He transposed the composition and finished it on three strings.

\* \* \* \* \*

That is living courageously—to have your "A" string snap and finish on three strings. It would have been exciting to hear Ole Bull with a perfect instrument. But it would have been more exciting to have heard him when the "A" string snapped and without self-pity he finished on three strings.

That is precisely what I propose to do. Wait for my body to repair itself, if it can. Regardless, *I will live life to the fullest,* healthy or sick, whole or in part. My "A" string has snapped. I intend to complete the concert of my life without it.

Success means different things to different people. We can be successful in one endeavor and fail in others. Few, if any, are successful in everything. I will never possess the physical strength I once had. Still, I can do many things without full strength.

Those of us who are handicapped can strive to reach the goal of overcoming our limitation. If that proves to be beyond our reach today, we can work to accommodate ourselves to live with the limitation. Robert Browning ingeniously wrote: "Ah, but a man's reach should exceed his grasp, or what's a heaven for?"

I applaud that strong individual determined enough to work until he has defeated his or her handicap. The real hero, however, is that dedicated soul, handicapped but joyful in life, even with a physical, mental, social, educational, or emotional limitation. *To take second best, and make something of it, is success!*

At the moment, I am a mind imprisoned in a body. No ordinary prison could keep me in the absolute confinement that has locked down virtually all my physical functions. I am sick, weak, helpless, powerless, unproductive, and utterly paralyzed. Though I do not want to admit it, I am overly anxious the majority of the time. Additionally, I constantly battle depression. In my heart of hearts I believe I will recover. However, I ponder the extent of my potential recovery.

Machines sustain me, nurses feed me, and a host of doctors are keeping me alive. I am one-hundred percent dependent on others. I am so far down, the only way I can go is up. It isn't possible to fall off the floor.

The question remains: Can I get up?

# One Thing after Another

*L*et's backtrack to when I am still very depressed and not feeling hopeful. Help is on the way. Bess asks two of my personal friends, Dr. Steve Yurco and Harold Riley, to give me a pep talk. They both readily agree to encourage me.

Dr. Yurco's visit is most meaningful, since he is not my physician. Steve tells me I *could* get well. Beyond that he tells me I *will* get well. I believe him, and think that is one reason I begin to recover. Never underestimate the value of a friend.

Harold Riley takes a different approach. He was in Philadelphia when his wife Dottie phoned to inform him of my illness. Harold told me, "In my hotel room, I prayed for you. You are going to get well. God told me you are going to get well!"

Helen Keller said: "If you have friends, you can endure anything." For the first time, on April 12, nine days after my paralysis, *I believe I will get well.* More importantly, I begin to want to get well. Up to this time, I am hoping God will let me die. Things appear hopeless. Death would be a welcome relief to the pain, helplessness, and frustration I am experiencing. Now, hope is emerging in my soul.

Never underestimate the power of friendship and prayer. More depressing experiences are ahead, but the assurance and prayers of these two men will help sustain me in down times. The words of these men are backed up by deeds in the ensuing months. Seldom does a day pass that one or both of them do not visit me. Always they assure me, "You will get well." Their encouragement is keeping me alive while the life-support systems are keeping my body alive.

A minister observes a man seated on a park bench who appears to be in dire circumstances. Wanting to help the man, the kind minister hands the transient a five-dollar bill. He whispers to the vagrant, "Never despair."

Passing by the tramp the following day, the minister is handed a roll of bills. Shocked the minister asks, "What is this?"

The transient replies, "Never Despair won the third race and paid eight-to-one!"

History records that when young Alexander the Great set out to conquer the known world, he led his armies over the Swiss Alps. He divested himself of all possessions.

His commanding officer said, "Sir, you have given away everything!"

Alexander replied, "We have kept hope. It is all we need."

\* \* \* \* \*

I still have hope. "Never Despair" is a good horse on which to ride. I keep reminding myself that I am on the bottom and can't fall off the floor. Things are good!

Things get even better. My wife and granddaughter Lisa visit me. They say, "Your spirits are better!" Both observe I am more relaxed. Lisa has a beautiful voice. She sings several hymns. As she sings "How Great Thou Art," tears are flowing down her sweet cheeks. Faith is growing. Hope is not dead. Tears fill my eyes and are rippling down my cheeks. Since I am unable to dry my own tears because of paralysis, Bess softly wipes them away.

The concert completed, Lisa informs me I have to live, so I can perform her wedding. That is pressure! I love all my grandchildren. Lisa, being my first grandchild, holds a special place in my heart.

Before Bess and Lisa depart, Sophia, my favorite nurse, enters the room. Sophia is a beautiful African-American. Her sweet smile and soft voice indicate a disposition that seemingly is always positive. Her concern is focused on the patient. She has the gift of anticipating my needs.

Whispering, she asks my wife if she can anoint me. She informs Bess, she has been praying I will recover. Aware I am a Baptist pastor, she knows my deep belief in the power of prayer.

Bess consents. Gently, Sophia places a drop of oil on my forehead. This is followed by one of the sweetest and strongest prayers I have ever heard. More important, God heard. That night I sleep soundly for the first time since entering the hospital.

It seems I have been in Seton Hospital's Critical Neurological Care Unit for a lifetime. It is April 13 and appears to be my lucky day. Bess phones at 8:00 a.m. and my nurse indicates I am stable. Later at 10:00 a.m. she comes to my room and observes, "You appear to be well rested." I want to say, "I should be. I have been in bed for a lifetime," but I cannot talk. My blood pressure and pulse are improved. Dr. Douglas is pleased and tells Bess I am where I should be at this time in my GBS.

New medication is given for my blood pressure. It is down to 85. Harold Riley and another good friend, Clyde Danks, come by to visit and encourage me. There is not a cloud in my sky. I have had two good days in a row.

In NCC one should not get overly excited when there are a couple of good days. Things can change in a hurry … and they do. I rest well during the night but awaken the following morning with a slight temperature of 100.4. My stomach is very swollen and my face is red and puffy. I am substantially more uncomfortable.

Morphine is started to ease my discomfort. The nurse suctions my lungs several times, extracting a vast amount of phlegm. My blood pressure has risen from 136 over 65 to 176 over 80. My pulse jumps from 83 to 90. My oxygen level, being constantly monitored, drops dramatically. Murphy's Law is, "If anything can go wrong, it will." I was sure proving Murphy right!

Dr. Shepherd, a pulmonary specialist, is summoned and visits me late in the evening. Nurses are being compelled to suction fluid from my lungs more frequently than they would like. My lungs, sustained by the respirator, are struggling with a fluid buildup from pneumonia. It seems they will never function perfectly.

My bowels are not working correctly. My stomach is distended. Dr. Joe Reneau, who for years was our family physician, tells Bess it is an ileus. Auxiliary illnesses from the GBS are increasing, causing this blockage of the intestine. What began as a good day has degenerated into one of deep discomfort.

When Bess arrives the next morning, nurses report I have gone through a very disagreeable night. That is an understatement. Sometime during the night, Dr. Shepherd is compelled to do a bronchostomy (the insertion of a tube into the lungs to suction fluids). Even with the regular suctioning done by the nurses, fluid is still building in my lungs, making breathing increasingly arduous.

My stomach continues to be severely swollen. The doctor reports to Bess, "Ralph's kidneys are not working properly and they are getting into trouble. This is a rare complication of IVGG treatment." Thank God he tells this to my wife, not me. Right now I do not need any more bad news … neither does she. I am just beginning to believe I will get well, but my confidence is weak. Serious illness can crush optimism. Many, if not most, GBS patients are despondent. At the moment I am one of the *many*.

Dr. Heinz, a urologist, is summoned to help. He increases my $H^2O$ intake. He reports to me that my kidneys are getting soft. Additionally, he suspects I have Clostridium Difficile. This disease is new to my limited medical vocabulary. I use the abbreviation Cdiff. It manifests itself with diarrhea, fever, and general discomfort. "Lousy" remains the word that best describes the way I feel.

Cdiff. is contagious. It is very transmittable. A sign is placed outside my door telling visitors they must wear gowns, caps, and gloves when entering the room. Isolation and hand washing are the primary means of preventing transmission. The Cdiff. spores can live five months in the environment unless they are removed physically with cleansing. The spores are picked up on hands from furniture and bathrooms, and transferred to the face and mouth. Since I cannot move my hands to transfer the spores, they have been delivered to my room by hospital personnel.

Swallowing even a single spore can "colonize" the intestines (gut). I am receiving many antibiotics. This has caused the normal germs in the intestines to be reduced or killed, which has allowed the Cdiff. to grow fast and take over. The result is a toxin that produces diarrhea and abdominal pain. Healthy people usually have no problem. Eventually the normal germs grow and the Cdiff. gets "crowded out."

This is my first encounter with Cdiff. It will not be my last. This disease will plague me in the coming months. I am in diapers … with diarrhea. Beyond this impairment, my fever is high. The hospital has a simple solution to prevent this disease: **Hand Washing!**

The problem is that hospital personnel do not wash their hands every time they enter or leave a patient's room. I understand. They are in and out of patients' rooms many times during the day. Each nurse has several patients. They are working under heavy pressure with emergencies occurring hourly. It is easy to forget, or neglect, to wash hands. I admire the nurses and hospital personnel. Nevertheless, my Cdiff. is probably a result of their carelessness.

A tube is inserted through my nose into my stomach to empty bile. I am a sad-looking patient. There is a tracheotomy tube in my throat, a tube in one nostril to feed me, and now a second tube in my other nostril to drain bile. They have attached a monitor to my finger, a blood pressure apparatus on my arm, heart-monitor cups on my chest, an IV in my other arm, and a catheter in my penis. The doctors and nurses have me drained, tubed, taped, monitored, and I am inert.

I have not lost my sense of humor. I ask Bess for a Diet Coke. These are the first words I have spoken since the tracheal tube was inserted. How I could whisper my request is a mystery. Since I cannot swallow, how would I drink it? Needless to say, I do not get the Coke.

It is Easter Sunday, April 16. I am resting well, though frustrated that I cannot lead the church in worship. This Sunday is the high point of the church year. No suctioning of my lungs is necessary. I am moving toward a good day.

My good Easter Sunday gets even better, as Bess visits me after attending church. She relates to me the associate pastor's sermon, then reads to me the record of Christ's resurrection from the Gospel of Matthew. Since I cannot hold a Bible, and thus cannot read my Bible, this is spiritually refreshing.

Then Bess reports that my doctor told his Sunday school class I would be out of NCC in ten days to two weeks. How wonderful! It is Easter, my sweet wife reads the Bible to me, and my doctor thinks I am getting stronger.

Two days later the medical team decides to put a catheter in my left shoulder. This surgical procedure places a tube into a major blood vessel, allowing the medical staff to give injections and draw blood. I am sedated and Dr. Bridges performs the surgery in my room. When the surgery is finished, I have no recollection of it. Heavy sedation keeps me in a mental fog the remainder of the day.

Now that I have a catheter in my shoulder, blood can be drawn from the catheter and medicine will be injected through the catheter. *No more injections in my arm!* That is wishful thinking. I find that two thirds of the nurses slip the needle into the catheter and medicate me. The other third either do not know I have a catheter, or prefer injecting me in my arm, butt, or elsewhere. It is explained to me that they can get a "clear" blood sample only by going through my vein. Some of the nurses do not know I have a catheter. Either they do not read my chart, or read it and do not care to use the catheter for injections.

The catheter is a good idea if the nurses: (A) know you have it and (B) choose to use it. As previously stated, I believe nurses love to slip a needle into a patient's skin.

April 19 finds me stable and unchanged. Dr. Douglas thinks he sees a bigger twitch in my right leg. My kidneys have not degenerated, but something is wrong with my gut. Dr. Williford gives me medication to stimulate my viscera. My nerve insulation is gone.

In spite of my weak physical condition, I am feeling much improved. I ask my wife for my mail, and inquire if she has paid the bills. I realize how inappropriate my question is. I am just making conversation. Bess is offended. In her view, I am questioning her ability to care for routine household affairs.

*Making conversation* is an incorrect phrase. With the tracheotomy tube stuck in my throat, I cannot speak. Bess and I can, however, communicate. One of our good nurses (or friends?) brings in a chart with the alphabet and a few simple requests written out. When Bess and I "talk" she points to letters in the alphabet; I blink my eyes at the correct letter, and after an extended period of time a word is spelled. This is the method employed in my "talking." On the following page is a replica of the chart:

## Front Side

A  B  C  D  E  F     SHEET
G  H  I  J  K  L     I'M HOT
M  N  O  P  Q  R     ICE          NURSE
S  T  U  V  W  X     T V         VASELINE
      Y  Z           RUB LEGS    HAND MOVED
                  READ          SUCTION
0  1  2  3  4  5  6  7  8  9    WET RAG     HEAD

The back side of this chart provided additional options. Here are my choices that could be understood with one eye blink for "yes" and two blinks for "no."

## Back Side

PLEASE TURN     ON/OFF     EYE GLASSES
TV     RADIO     LIGHTS     MOUTH CARE
_____     _____

PLEASE     ELEVATE/LOWER     VISITORS YES/NO
MY HEAD     MY LEGS     _____
_____     PLEASE LET ME SLEEP

PLEASE BRING BLANKET     _____
_____     BRING SLEEPING PILL

PLEASE TURN ME     _____
_____     NEED PAIN MEDICATION

PLEASE STRAIGHTEN BED     _____
_____     PAIN LEVEL:

YES/NO     1 2 3 4 5 6 7 8 9 10
_____     _____

ROOM:     I'M THIRSTY
TOO WARM    TOO COLD     I'M NAUSEATED

# *Anything That Can Go Wrong, Probably Will*

$\mathcal{I}$f the sea of life is calm, it will inevitably get stormy. Late this night two nurses turn me in bed. They fail to notice the tracheotomy tube has slipped out of my throat. All my vital statistics immediately drop. I gasp for breath! Since I cannot talk, I am incapable of telling them of my condition. I am helpless. I am unable to breathe without the respirator. I am dying!

My sense of humor steps forward. I remember that I have seen more people die in the hospital than anywhere else. This is not consoling. It is dangerous to be in the hospital!

Somehow I do what I cannot do. I cry out loudly, "My throat hurts!" With my spoken word the nurses realize the tracheotomy tube is not in my throat. They panic. I am getting drowsy, and slipping into a trance. The nurse monitoring my status outside the room is alerted by the beeping monitor alarm. Her routine job has suddenly become exciting. The last thing I recall is seeing her jump from her tall stool and bolt toward the door.

Everything is black, total darkness. I am in another dimension. The next several minutes of my life are blank. It is as if someone turned off the light inside me. There is neither pain nor panic. Peace floods my mind. Totally helpless, I am completely relaxed. This must be the feeling a dying person has when he or she steps into eternity. The Bible refers to death as falling asleep. That accurately describes my experience.

Business picks up in my room. They call a **CODE STAT**. Nurses run from all units in Neurological Critical Care. A doctor rushes into my room. My heart has stopped beating! Silence! Darkness! Lifeless! *I am dead!*

My wife is in the hall. She had left the room, while the nurses were turning me and caring for my personal needs. Hearing the alarm on my monitors, seeing the nurses running into my room, and witnessing the arrival of a new doctor, she knows I am in serious trouble.

Things become more intense when the hospital chaplain comes to be with her. The lady chaplain asks Bess, "Can I help you?"

Bess replies, "No."

The chaplain walks away. With the chaplain exiting, Bess sits outside my room and waits alone. Often I have pondered why the chaplain departed, or why the chaplain did not pray with my wife. Bess is alone. My status is questionable. Code Stat means **SERIOUS.**

Within minutes the doctor might come to Bess and say, "Sorry, he died …"

And the chaplain left …

Skillfully working on me, the doctor stimulates my heart and starts its beat. After ten minutes the nurses give my wife the high sign, thumbs up. To this day I do not know the name of the doctor who saved my life. Doctors and nurses are the unsung heroes of our generation. To the unknown doctor and nurses who saved my life, "Thank You!"

My heart did stop beating for a few seconds (or minutes). For whatever time, I was physically dead. No sane person wants to experience heart failure. The occurrence is never forgotten. Normally, it is not a round-trip.

The best-known passage of Scripture in the Bible is Psalm 23. They tell me David wrote the 23rd Psalm. I could have written it. He just beat me to it! "Yea, though I walk through the valley of the shadow of death, I will fear no evil for Thou art with me …" That was my experience, no fear and perfect peace. It is like something I have experienced every night of my life, sleep. One moment I am alert, the next instant … nothingness.

My blood pressure is abnormally high, 240 over 115. By 10:30 this evening, my blood pressure returns to normal. With the adrenaline rush, it is 1:00 a.m. before I finally fall asleep. This episode nearly sent me into a permanent slumber.

Early in my illness, death is what I desired. With this experience my outlook decidedly changes. Desperately I want to get well. I am still uncertain whether I can, or will, heal but the desire to heal becomes the driving force in my life.

In the days following, I ride on an emotional roller coaster. Crying has become a part of my daily routine. The doctor tells the family this is normal with nerve disorder illness. I am very despondent. I look away or down when people talk to me. I can't move my head, but I avoid eye contact. The family believes I am depressed. I disagree. They are probably correct, but I believe I am on the *edge* of depression. I have not completely walked into that dark, mysterious abyss.

It is my understanding there are two types of depression: situational and chemical. Situational depression relates to circumstances that overwhelm the individual. Chemical depression occurs when, due to body chemistry, the neurons in the brain do not quickly or adequately connect. At the moment I am a candidate for both kinds of depression, but have neither.

The family, nurses, and doctors have every right to believe I am depressed. My complaint is, "It is too hot!"

Then within minutes, "It is too cold!" I want therapy, but when the nurses move me preparing for therapy, I protest. Nothing pleases me.

Perhaps you wonder, "How can you complain? You have a tracheotomy tube in your throat." True. I protest with my eyes. They express the emotions in my soul. Nurses report to Bess my *eye talk*. They interpret *eye talk* to be complaining.

Nurses are professionals, and are not supposed to be that sensitive. If they know I am complaining, which I am not, they should attempt to alleviate my pain. They don't. They simply report my belligerence to my wife. All this accomplishes is to upset her, and further frustrate me. With my frustration, nothing makes me content.

To compound my misery, the nurses decide I should sit in a special chair thirty or more minutes, several times a day. With great effort the nursing staff places me in the special chair. I hate it! Ten minutes pass, and I am grumbling. Grumbling is not the correct word because I have the tracheotomy tube in my throat and cannot talk. The best I can do to protest is frown with my eyes. This is not getting much attention, or response, from the nurses.

By April 27 the nurses have me sitting in the special chair regularly. On that infamous day those mean nurses, after plotting with my wife, put me in the chair and walk out of the room. For the longest thirty-five minutes of my life, I sit upright in mortal suffering.

Even hurt can help! This becomes the first step in getting me to sit upright on my own. It is, I will later learn, the introduction to my rehabilitation. How can sitting in a chair, with so much pain and frustration, be so important? It taught me an invaluable lesson regarding rehabilitation. *Rehabilitation will cause pain. I must ignore or overcome discomfort and pain if I want to successfully rehabilitate. My discomfort and pain will become the pathway to healing and restoration.*

Naturally, this causes my blood pressure to remain high. They give me Procardia. The blood pressure stays high. More Procardia is administered with no positive result. Dr. Herford is notified. After examination he becomes greatly concerned, telling the nurses to monitor me even more closely. My vital signs are pointing to disaster.

The next morning the nurses decide to give me a rest from the feeding tube by removing it from my nose. Apparently the tube is clogged from the formula they are feeding me. This proves to be a major mistake, even though by evening I am looking and feeling much better. When the nurses try to reinsert the nose-feeding tube, they cannot. They give it their best effort, off and on, for two very long hours. My throat is swollen. The nose and throat passage is too narrow. Irritation has my throat red, raw, and swollen.

Three hours later a nose-and-throat doctor reinserts the tube through my nose into my stomach. I am under heavy sedation. This procedure proves to be very difficult and takes an hour. In the process, the tube is moved from my left nostril to the right. An x-ray reveals the new tube extending into my stomach is correctly placed.

Because of the three-hour process, my blood pressure rises even higher. With that my pulse is extremely rapid. The old ship of my body is listing badly. I am wondering if the medical team can plug all the leaks in this "Titanic."

Dr. Douglas tells my wife I am very stubborn, and I want everything explained to me. How right he is! He goes on to say, if he explained, I would not understand. And besides, he did not have time to explain. His medical skills are terrific. He needs to work on his communication and bedside techniques. They need a lot of help.

Had I been able to talk, I would have explained to my good doctor that "knowledge is power." Even a brief explanation would be of great comfort to me. Physical body healing is connected to the mind. Being a neurologist, I presume, Dr. Douglas knows mind and body are inseparably connected.

My GBS nerve damage has caused facial paralysis of the left side of my mouth, lip, and chin. Realizing this, I conjecture I am growing weaker, not stronger.

Furthermore, I am still having difficulty with my respiratory therapy. Beyond that, mucus is coming out of my nose. Respiratory therapist Charlie Burke attempts to suction my throat. The staff works diligently trying to disengage me from the respirator. For ten minutes I breathe on my own, without the ventilator. This is a significant milestone. It indicates my lung muscles and nerves are operative.

The new strategy is to take me off the respirator every two hours. After three attempts, this scheme is temporarily abandoned. My blood pressure severely elevates when I am not on the respirator. Weakness of lung nerves remains a major problem.

My breathing parameters are presently 400. When they reach 1000, I can be off the respirator. Dr. Denton tells me I am not ready to breathe on my own. All the doctors, however, believe I am progressing. At 400, needing to be at 1000, I have reached 40 percent of the goal.

I realize I am still on a downhill slide. When Bess visits all I do is mouth, "I want to go home." It is April 25 and I have been in NCC twenty-five days. Immobilized, twenty-five days in NCC is a lifetime.

My throat is bleeding because I have been on the tracheotomy tube so long. Dr. Leary believes it is an irritation caused by so much suctioning. With my blood pressure rising to 200 over 101, they will not give physical therapy, or even allow me to sit in the chair to strengthen my back. No longer do they take me off the respirator, even for short spans. My blood pressure remains too high.

We receive more bad news as Dr. Shapiro tells Bess the daily x-rays indicate my right lung looks exceptionally bad. At 5:30 a.m. he has to perform another bronchoscopy. The lungs are saturated. My pulse and blood pressure both drop dramatically. The good news is he removes several plugs blocking my lungs.

My heart stops again. The nurses bag me. Providentially available, Dr. Watts handles the emergency. This good doctor, whom I have never met, saves my life. This is my second death experience. Again, everything goes black. It is like dimming a light until there is total darkness. Only the expertise of Dr. Watts awakens me, and returns my life.

Later in the evening my blood pressure drops to 60. Dr. Denton has to do another bronchoscopy early the following morning. The lower half of my right lung remains clogged. After the bronchoscopy, suctioning is occurring nearly every hour. Miserable, distressed, disconsolate, and in agony are inadequate terms to describe my plight. To make matters worse, Dr. Helmer tells Bess I will possibly be in NCC another month or six weeks.

Once again my resolve to live is weakening. Normally, I am an optimist. In my mind I keep listing my challenges: totally paralyzed, on a respirator, an uncomfortable catheter, wearing diapers, fed through a nose tube, Gushong in left shoulder, oxymeter on my finger, peripheral nerves useless, extreme high blood pressure, hurting with every touch. I am pondering if I can continue to live in this tortured, helpless, frustrating condition. Keeping a will to live is almost impossible … almost, not totally.

Bess, who knows me better than I know myself, senses how discouraged I am. When I mouth "take me home," tears fill her beautiful eyes. Later she tells me, "That almost killed me." She holds my lifeless hand and asks me not to give up. I tell her I will not give up. That is a promise I try desperately to keep. Still things are at a low ebb.

Miserable best describes my condition. I am crushed and broken-hearted.

When Bess leaves in the evening, plagued with the GBS and its complications, I am thinking, *Everything is bad. No, that is not true. Nothing is all wrong. Even a clock that has stopped running is right twice a day. I can see, hear, sleep, blink my eyes. … I am still alive!*

Moreover, my wife and family are staying right by my side. A few good friends visit often. I have dedicated doctors, nurses, and attendants who are working around the clock to help me overcome this illness.

The first fifteen days of May are rocky. Dr. Douglas tells Bess there has been major nerve damage which may take years to repair. Tests reveal practically no nerve response There could be some residual paralysis. Bess has a good long cry.

One of my wife's strongest attributes is her honesty. She and I have always been truthful in our marriage. Thus she feels compelled to share with me our doctor's evaluation and prognosis. As tactfully as possible, Bess shares the medical report. Unable to talk, the best I can, I assure her we will cope with whatever the future holds.

*Things are not as bad as they seem! They could be worse! They will get better! I can't fall off the floor. It still works for me!*

Dr. Clark frequently performs bronchoscopies. The ventilator tube keeps popping out of my throat. Nurses are suctioning my lungs every two hours, or less. My stomach is distended again. In spite of the illnesses, the medical team tries to wean me off the urine catheter. This is unsuccessful.

Only two things go well. Room oxygen is 20 percent. I am able to breathe on 30 percent oxygen. I am two thirds of the way to escaping from dependence on the respirator. This indicates major breathing progress. Second, I manage to send my wife flowers twice during these fifteen days. She is the love of my life. If possible, my illness is harder on her than on me. Pressure is nearly unbearable on a wife when her husband is critically ill. Without a doubt, family members need more support than the patient.

# Hallucinations and Annoyances

*M*y sixth week in NCC brings a new challenge. When Bess visits I tell her that nurses are sleeping under my bed, and in my bed. It is evident she does not believe me. This makes me irate. I request she ask my son to visit me. When Wallace arrives I tell him four nurses were in bed with me the previous night. Moreover, a nurse with her baby is sleeping under my bed at night. This is as real to me as life itself. He patiently and sympathetically listens. It is obvious he does not believe a word I am saying.

When he departs, I weep. Neither my wife nor son believe me. My next request is that they tell my doctor. All this is painful. I can't talk and am spelling out the story on the alphabet chart. What is factual to me is fantasy to my wife, son, and doctor. They refuse to believe me. I am exhausted trying to communicate using the spell chart.

Our neurologist, Dr. Marledge, tells Bess that for rest, instead of Atavan, they gave me Restoril, and I hallucinated. Vancomycin is administered again that afternoon, and by evening I am totally confused. For example, I have very little hair. I tell Dr. Joe Reneau, however, to "hold the comb." The nurses explain to Bess that confusion goes along with a lengthy stay in critical care. It is obvious to everyone but me—I am confused.

More confusion follows. I tell Dr. Marledge that at night I can move my hands and even hold and read the paper. When morning comes, however, I can't move them. Moreover, I tell my wife and doctor I got up at night and used the bathroom. Since neither believes me, I decide not to tell them this happened in New York!

I am in Fantasy Land.

My daughter Diane spends the night with me. She is humoring me. It works! No nurses in my bed this night. I do wake up at midnight to tell her I am going to *walk* to the bathroom. I am still in Fantasy Land. On May 28, I tell the nurses I am tied down to the bed and to please untie me. How foolish! Why tie down a totally paralyzed person? My reasoning ability is impaired. Logic has fled and has been replaced by an overactive imagination.

These hallucinations continue for several weeks. One night I imagine I see two nurses sleeping on a picture frame that hangs on the wall in front of my bed. When I start to relay this happening, I pause, then stop, realizing how foolish the story sounds. This dream or fantasy is so outlandish, it convinces me I am hallucinating. Eventually the hallucinations cease.

* * * * *

Persistence pays big dividends. On May 28, Bess observes me slightly moving my shoulder. My body *is* rebuilding itself. The doctor sees my chest move. I am able to sit in the chair for forty-five minutes. The respiration therapist reports I now breathe spontaneously twice with one assist. Dr. Douglas believes I am stronger. I am moving my fingers slightly. This is progress!

With all the sickness-healing, living-dying occupying the doctors, nurses, and family, I am having three small annoyances. They begin with flowers.

Many people express concern regarding my GBS. Bess receives over six-thousand cards and letters. Some people are gracious enough to send flowers. We are deeply grateful and humbled by the concern and prayers of these sweet people. Normally flowers are not permitted in NCC. One bouquet is so beautiful that a nurse sits it in the windowsill of my room. The flowers bring brightness to the room and happiness to my heart.

One of my more frustrating nights is the second evening the flowers are in my room. Late in the evening, when I am nearly asleep, a gnat decides to roost in my ear. He flies around my earlobe, lands, then continues to make these round-trips in and out of my ear. Unable to move, I cannot swat the gnat. I now have a better understanding of the phrase "weak as a gnat." The gnat may be weak, but he is stronger than I! Having no way to alert a nurse, my ear and I endure the gnat most of the night. The next morning Bess has the beautiful flowers removed, solving the gnat problem.

The second annoyance is a friendly mosquito. Why the mosquito decides to enter NCC, I will never know. She doesn't seem ill. But, she leaves healthier, after dining on my blood all evening. My hatred for insects intensifies. This episode is my most helpless feeling ever. Being chewed on by a mosquito and being unable to do anything about it is frustration at the highest level.

The third annoyance is bizarre. I awaken one morning with several whelps on my back and posterior. The nurses are perplexed as to the cause. With my nerve problem and the sedation I am being given, I am unaware of the red spots on my body.

When the nurses talk with Bess, they tell her of the mysterious red spots. Realizing it is external and knowing my backside is affected, Bess scours the room. What is the cause? In the window sill she finds a small colony of ants. Ants have invaded my room! Under the bed she finds more of the insects. Several of them apparently decided to sleep with me.


Dr. David Livingston was a dedicated medical missionary. His life was spent in Central Africa. He charted out the headwaters of the

Nile River and sent the maps to England, which resulted in the black slave trade being stamped out in Africa. He was honored by England as one of her most revered citizens. His heart is buried in Africa. His body is buried in Westminster Abbey. When asked to return his body to England, the natives agreed but said his heart would remain with them. Thus the natives cut the heart from his dead body and lovingly buried it in Africa.

A visitor once asked Dr. Livingston if the lions, tigers, elephants, and other animals threatened him. "No," he responded, "but the chiggers nearly drive me crazy."

I resonate with that. The gnats, mosquitoes, and ants are maddening to me.

Thank God, April and May have passed! It is June 1, and the therapist takes the ventilator tube from my throat, placing a CPAP in the hole in my throat. This device plugs up the throat opening and allows me to breathe on my own. My heart is beating rapidly. I am excited and fearful at the same time. Excited because the CPAP allows me to talk, and fearful I can't breathe, since I am no longer on the respirator.

What do you say after being mute for two months? My first words are to my precious wife, who stands by my side so faithfully. With great effort, I softly say, "I love you." Tears fill her eyes, and mine. Now I can verbally communicate for brief periods of time each day. This is my most noteworthy progress thus far. **I can finally talk!**

Have you noticed; as soon as one problem is solved another appears? That is one way to describe life—facing a problem and solving it, only to be challenged with another. The only place where everything appears completely organized all the time is the cemetery. Having problems indicates we are alive and well.

Wallace E. Johnson, cofounder of Holiday Inns of America, once told me that there are no problems, only opportunities. At this point in my illness God is giving me too many opportunities. A few less *opportunities* would be a welcome relief.

I am challenged with another problem, I mean opportunity. Something has gone wrong with the nose-feeding tube that extends into my stomach. The doctor has to reinsert the tube further because I have food in my mouth. Since the first day of my illness on April 4, not one morsel of food has entered my mouth. All feeding has been through tubes in my nose or arm. But somehow I have food in my mouth. … How did this happen?

My breathing is rapid and shallow. This forces the pulmonary doctor to raise the oxygen flow to 50 percent. Dr. Douglas, sensing Bess is discouraged, states, "He will take two steps forward and one step backward." With the reverse progress I am encountering, Dr. Douglas' remark is encouraging to my wife. Moreover, the statement proves to be entirely accurate. I burn *"two steps forward and one step backward"* into my mind. In some of my toughest moments this self-evident truth will keep me going. It works in reverse, too: *if I take a step backward, I will take two steps forward!*

Retreat has never been in my vocabulary. I never enjoyed walking backwards. John Bunyon wrote of a character named "Mr. Facing-Both-Ways." He faced one direction and rowed his boat in the opposite way. Hopefully, I am facing and walking in the direction of restoration. I deeply desire to be salubrious. Before I am sound as a bell, progress will be two steps forward and one step backward. There are no reverse gears in life, but there are reverse gears in the healing process.

One positive benefit of my illness is that I have lost forty-eight pounds. For health's sake no one seems concerned about my weight loss. The nurses are concerned that I sleep too much. They feel I am depressed. My response is, "What else can I do?" Totally paralyzed, on a respirator, constantly hurting, makes depression and sleep appealing as escape mechanisms. It is the only thing I do well.

My mind is still confused. I tell Bess my bed split in two. I also imagine I walk to the bathroom, but someone has moved it. In my mind I know I can get out of bed and walk across the room to a chair without any assistance. In reality I can't. The doctors are increasing the drugs, and I am increasingly confused.

This reminds me about the ninety-year-old lady who had a baby. When a ninety-year-old has a baby, it is news! The local television crew comes to interview her. They ask if they can see the baby. She replies, "Yes, as soon as the baby cries."

"Why do you want us to wait until the baby cries?" They inquire.

"Because I forgot where I put him."

I understand! Day by day in NCC, I am getting more confused. Dr. Helmer suggests I read books. Hurting, and being unable to hold a book, or even turn a page, I am not interested or able to read a book. It is, however, a great idea.

My doctor is accurate. My mind needs exercise. It should move from my state of ill health to something constructive, positive, and encouraging. Self-talk has always been a vital part of my life. So, I have conversations with myself. Since I cannot speak audibly, I do it in my mind. Additionally, I quote to myself everything I have memorized. Working on exercising my mind, I begin to recall my childhood, high school, and college days. I reflect on my marriage, children, vacations, pleasant times, and friends. This proves to be refreshing and inspirational. It seems infinitely better than reading a book, or having someone read to me.

Recalling literature I have memorized proves exceptionally helpful. For example, I remember the passages memorized from Shakespeare's plays:

> *To be or not to be, that is the question, ...*
> *All the world's a stage ... one man playing seven parts ...*

My mind recalls passages by William Wordsworth memorized in high school:

> *I wandered lonely as a cloud, that floats on high over hill and dale,*
> *When all at once I saw a crowd, a host of golden daffodils.*

Most helpful of all are precious promises from the Bible:

> *The Lord is my shepherd, I shall not want ...*
> *I will never leave you nor forsake you ...*
> *Fear not for I am with you, be not dismayed ...*

That is what I am, and where I am, "dismayed." Thinking of playing my part, seeing daffodils, and knowing God is with me, lifts the cloud from my confused mind. I am certainly not the most intelligent person, but talking to myself helps free my mind of its confused state. Self-talk can be positive, encouraging, and healing.

I recall reading of two men who were in prison looking outside from their cells on a dark night; one prisoner saw the *bars* while the other saw the *stars*. My self-talk, mind games, and recalling memorized scripture and poetry helps me see the bright future, not the dismal present. My doctor's book idea is wonderful. I have translated it into my own *Book of Life*. Humor is also playing a vital role in my recovery. Laughter has healing power.

Once again I am on the road to recovery!

The physical therapist observes I am having less pain with my exercises. I am indeed feeling better. I even ask Bess to read me *USA Today*. Shrugging my shoulders, moving my stomach muscles, and twitching my left thigh and upper arm are signs of minuscule progress. Most important, I am off the respirator and on the CPAP all day! The following day is even better. I am able to sit in the chair 50 minutes. For an hour I am off all breathing support. My lungs, muscles, and nerves are being restored!

I am on a mountaintop about to fall. The next day I have diarrhea. This is not a touch of diarrhea, but a constant flow. Since I am still in diapers, this is a challenging problem for the nurses. My frustration level is 100 percent.

I am like the man who said to his friend, "My bowels are locked. I go to the bathroom all day long."

The friend responded, "You have diarrhea, your bowels are not locked."

The sick man responded, "My bowels are locked ... in the open position."

Late in the afternoon Dr. Shapiro takes my wife into the hall to express his concern. He states, "There is no improvement in Ralph's breathing." (This isn't exactly accurate.) He goes on to explain that my breathing is shallow. (This is accurate.) He sees more months of slow improvement and many months of rehab with no guarantees. He indicates that the family needs to look into other places to keep me since my insurance will not pay for NCC much longer.

When Bess returns to the room after talking with Dr. Shapiro, using the spell chart I ask what he said. Bess responds, "They will give you four more months on the respirator. If you are not off it by then, they will need to put you in a nursing home."

My response is that I am beginning to realize I am not going to get well. However, I will not quit fighting.

My sweet wife prays with me and leaves. She writes in the record she is keeping, "I had prayer with him and left in a broken heap ... and alone."

It is June 12. Exactly forty-four years ago, Bess and I were married. This day will pass without my even realizing it is our anniversary. Bess does not mention it, fearing I will worry. She is right, I would have worried. It is not a happy anniversary, but a sad one. Bess informs me no one in Austin has been on a ventilator so long with so little progress. Depression has set in and all I want to do is sleep. The doctors are not talking to us. Their silence is shouting, "Things are not well."

A new treatment is instituted to improve my breathing. I attempt to breathe through a straw measuring air pressure. The nurses appear pleased with the result. I am placed on the CPAP for two hours. Amazingly, the next day Dr. Douglas reports my breathing and diaphragm muscles are greatly improved. Also, shoulder shrugs are stronger and hands are more supple. He is still concerned there is major damage to extremities, since I have been paralyzed so long.

My wife writes in her diary, "Lord, help us!" Little did we know how much He would.

My NCC nurses are suffering from burnout. Care is not good. I go for days without getting my teeth brushed. Unless the alarm on the respirator goes off, no one checks on me. Often I am wet with sweat because of too much cover. At times I am cold with too little cover. The good nurses are used to having patients a few hours, or days. Now they have faithfully nursed me 70 days, and progress is remarkably slow. Were I a nurse, I would be discouraged and disinterested, too. I would wonder if patient Ralph Smith will ever leave.

The doctors are getting testy with my wife. They are receiving inquiries from our health insurance carrier. One doctor suggests I be moved to a nursing home. Though I am showing improvement, it is painfully slow. I understand everyone's frustration with my slow progress. I am the most frustrated of all!

Another personal crisis has arisen. For four years I have served as chairman of the building committee for the new headquarters building of the Home Mission Board of the Southern Baptist Convention (now the North American Mission Board). We had purchased thirty-four acres of choice land just outside Atlanta, Georgia, from Ross Perot, Jr. Plans were drawn for the new headquarters building, contracts were signed, and now our twenty-five-million-dollar project is completed. As building committee chairman, I am to participate in the dedication and opening of the new headquarters building. This is to occur when the Southern Baptist Convention meets in Atlanta.

It is painfully obvious I can't attend the dedication and opening of the new facility. Mrs. Linda Bennett, my secretary, comes to NCC and I dictate a message of congratulations to the Board. My precious daughter, Diane Love, volunteers to attend the dedication, offer my regrets for being absent, and read my greeting and congratulations at the dedication.

Later, I am told Diane did a superb job. I knew she would. Like father, like daughter! Not really—all her good traits are inherited from her mother. I supplied all her weaknesses.

I recall one day Bess caught our son Wallace jumping up and down on our bed. Correcting him she said, "If you don't stop jumping up and down on our bed, I am going to get a belt and spank you. Beds are not meant for jumping, but for sleeping."

With a mournful look he responded, "And belts are for holding up our pants, not for spanking little boys."

That moment I knew he would be a lawyer.

My mind journeys from reality to confusion. I ask the nurse for a pen to write a letter. With compassion she informs me I am immobile. Paralyzed so long, I have forgotten I am disabled. Moreover, I continue to dream I am living in an apartment in New York. Reality is hard to grasp. Psychologically I am being affected. Three months in NCC is having a crippling effect on my mind.

Once again I am reminded I must exercise my brain in a positive way. Reality must be mentally accepted, with optimism as my long-term approach. The greatest battle in overcoming my paralysis is not in strengthening and exercising limbs, but rather in sustaining a positive mind-set. Belief in a venture is infinitely more important than the facts.

Long before a paralyzed person can walk, he or she must believe it will happen. An old axiom is: "What the mind can conceive and believe—the mind can achieve." Of course, there are exceptions, but this self-help proverb is ordinarily true. My task is to force my mind to see me walking, traveling, and enjoying a normal life.

Most nurses are competent and gentle. Unfortunately, I have one nurse who is neither. On this day Perla, my most merciless nurse, decides to squeeze me into a stiff, tight, rubber vest to aid my breathing. She calls it uncomfortable. I call it torture. To make matters worse, the nurses sit me in the uncomfortable chair and depart from my room. After the longest 45 minutes of my life, they return and put me in bed.

Because of this unnecessary, stupid, and pointless treatment I am agitated. My blood pressure becomes highly elevated. I am depressed. Once again it is clearly demonstrated to me that I have no control over anything. The nurses, even without a doctor's directive, can and will do what they desire. When the family visits in the evening, I have withdrawn and do not respond to their conversation. I am helpless and have been mismanaged by an overzealous nurse.

It is my seventy-ninth day in NCC. Again fluid is building up in my lungs. The doctor performs another bronchoscopy to clean out plugs in my lungs. During the procedure I become sick at my stomach, because the nurses do not stop feeding me early enough before the bronchoscopy. Even in NCC, competent nurses and good doctors make mistakes. Only problem is, the patient is the one who suffers. I am the patient!

This mistake results in my having to stay on the respirator all day. My spirits are low and I am frustrated. My trachea is bleeding. I have been on the respirator so long, my throat has gotten soft and the tracheotomy tube is leaking. Dr. Myers is summoned to replace the tube.

The next day I am sleepy and nonresponsive. During the procedure yesterday, I was given too much sedation. During my lifetime I have taken few drugs. Consequently, when a normal dosage is given to me, it is usually an excess. Additionally, I have developed a staph infection around my trachea. My slight temperature is making me extremely uncomfortable.

Two days later I continue to feel lousy. My sewing machine is out of thread. I am a few fries short of a "happy meal." I am sleepy and refuse to take therapy. The nurses appear concerned. Since my pulse is 114, they keep me on the respirator all day. Looking into my wife's beautiful eyes, I spell out "I am tired of fighting." I have been in NCC two-and-a-half months with little or no progress. My temperature is 101 degrees. By drawing blood samples from my arm, not the shoulder catheter, the nurses make me more downcast.

Again the doctors start antibiotics. This drives my temperature down. By nightfall I am feeling better for two reasons. First, medically the antibiotics administered are effective in fighting the infection. Second, Dr. Charlie Felger comes by and assures me the GBS will not kill me. He refreshes my soul. Though not one of my attending physicians, he helps me immensely by his bright spirit and encouraging words. Medicine can touch the body, but it takes a friend to reach the heart and soul.

The next day, June 24, I manage to sit up in the chair for fifty minutes. This is significant because I am in good spirits when they place me back in bed. Fifty minutes is too long. My pulse elevates to 101 and I am forced to stay on the respirator for twelve hours. The next day I am so exhausted I remain on the ventilator all day. My body is rebelling.

I perceive my rehab is mismanaged, but I do not know why. Later I will learn that when one has GBS, exercise needs to be stopped *before the patient reaches the point of exhaustion.* They should have put me in the chair no longer than fifteen or twenty minutes, two or three times a day. Keeping me in the chair for fifty minutes is counterproductive. It does not make me stronger, but weakens me.

It seems that experience is something you do not get until just after you need it.

My exhaustion fuels my depression. Dr. Mazza prescribes Prozac. I am uncooperative and complaining. Specifically I do not like my therapist, Karen. She just does not know how to exercise a GBS patient. I believe I need stretching and passive exercise. She does neither. I am sure she is competent; however, I am hurting and exhausted. Another therapist is assigned to help me.

Bess gives me a pep talk. I consider it a lecture. Quickly I become angry. She is right—I need to be tough and accept therapy. Her encouragement helps, her lecture doesn't. I sit in the chair without complaint. Instead of taking me to the gym, the new therapist comes to my room. Scheduling of the gym is a problem, which is upsetting to me. My schedule is random. Therapy is necessary, and the therapist will not stick to a regular schedule.

Again my temperature is high. The nurses have to stick me three times to draw blood. Finally, they take it from a vein in my hand. My blood vessels do not appreciate being pierced with a needle. I am thinking the shoulder catheter could have been used rather than my vein. Tests reveal a staph infection in my blood causing my elevated stress level.

On June 29, I am on Vancomycin and totally confused. I tell my family the car keys are in my bed and there are twenty-five magazines stacked under the covers. My lungs are being suctioned every two or three hours. Green gook is coming from my lungs. My temperature remains elevated. Life is no fun. My driving desire is to get well! It appears I won't.

Everything I do seems to result in failure. So what, failure is no big deal! I did not learn to swim the first time I tried. I did not balance perfectly the first time I attempted to ride a bike. I did not hit the ball, the first time I swung a bat. Success is getting up one more time than you fall down. Babe Ruth struck out 1,330 times, but we remember the 714 home runs he hit. I've read that R. H. Macy failed seven times before his store in New York became a retail powerhouse.

Failure is often simply the prelude to the magnificent concert of achievement. So on the last day of June, Dr. Douglas observes a stronger shoulder shrug. He sees a twitch in my right arm, rotation in both legs and hip, and flex in my right foot. When he relates the good news I respond, "Dr. Douglas, that is the first positive statement you have made in three months."

Do not expect much encouragement from a neurologist. They are highly trained doctors, not cheerleaders. They dispense medicine, not pep talks. Without Dr. Douglas and his associates, I would already be dead. In spite of his pessimism, I admire Dr. Douglas and his associates. Ever so slowly, they are leading me out of this forest of Guillian-Barrè Syndrome. One bright day, I will walk!

The next day Dr. Mazza examines me. He says I can probably get off the respirator now; if, however, I develop a plug in my lungs and cannot cough it up, I will be in a life-threatening situation. He adds, "It could be fatal." His final words are, "Be patient, the day will come." He does not know what a short supply of patience I have left.

Karen, returning as my physical therapist, visits me on July 1, and discusses the exercises I need. My spirits are up. I am eager to go forward with therapy. She asks Bess to return in the afternoon to learn to help me with some of the exercises. When they leave I am in a humorous mood and stick out my tongue at both of them. Bess goes into the hall and has a good cry.

My sense of humor is helping me but hurting her. I am teasing. She imagines I am serious. Hospital business is no laughing matter.

I learn patients should not joke with hospital personnel, doctors, and especially with family. Bess is under a terrific strain. I should be more considerate. Humor, however, has kept me sane in this mysterious illness. Anxiety continues to plague me. I remain camped on the border of total depression.

Whatever I am doing is inadequate. Dr. Hudson arranges for the EMG test to measure my muscle reaction. There is little improvement. However, I can now sit in the chair without great pain. Prozac is discontinued, causing my spirit to be lifted, perhaps due to decreased medication. I am in the same pattern of something bad, followed by something good, followed by something bad. It is two steps forward and one backward, as Dr. Douglas predicted.

The medical team continues to wean me off the respirator. My oxygen content is reduced to 35 percent. The respiration therapist plans to try oxygen with no pressure from the respirator. Good plan, but it does not work. On July 5, I flunk the breathing test again. Nurses hoped I could be off the respirator thirty minutes. I last ten. The timing is bad. I have been sitting in the chair for thirty minutes, which is very tiring. Currently, breathing requires tremendous concentration and energy.

Regardless of my failure, Dr. Morledge, Dr. Douglas' partner, is pleased with my progress. I am allowed to sleep the remainder of the day.

The day of rest gives me new strength. I sit in the chair twice on July 6 and I stay on the CPAP all day with little difficulty. It is obvious I am making progress and my attitude is greatly improved. Dr. Morledge's encouragement has given me renewed hope.

# Misery and Miracles

From the onset of my GBS, I am assured by physicians, nurses, friends, and family I will recover, if I do not die in the process. This enigmatic statement means GBS usually does not kill the patient. Its side illnesses may kill the patient. Medical studies indicate less than five percent of GBS patients die from the syndrome.

I continue to struggle with varied and different illnesses that are side effects from the GBS. Pneumonia attacks my lungs. My doctors help me rid myself of pneumonia. Almost immediately, I develop a kidney problem. That being cured, I contact Cdiff. with high fever, diarrhea, and chills. Meanwhile, my lungs are opened and closed by a respirator. The suctioning of my lungs by the staff has me in a life-and-death struggle to breathe, and to keep my lungs from filling with fluid. I have one anxiety attack after another. These attacks elevate my blood pressure and pose the risk of a heart attack or stroke.

Nevertheless, during all this process of bouncing from one illness to another, my body *is* rebuilding itself. There can be progress, when seemingly there is none.

\* \* \* \* \*

For example, at the speed of 1,000 miles an hour, our planet rotates. We are on this giant spaceship, Earth, traveling around the Sun at 66,000 miles an hour. Without our realizing it, day and night, we are traveling at the speed of 67,000 miles an hour!

The myelin sheath around my nerves is slowly being rebuilt. Though I am fragile, and outwardly there is little to indicate progress, inwardly my body is miraculously rebuilding.

My progress is such that the hospital sends Lorraine Stewart, a speech therapist, to teach me how to eat. *How unnecessary*, I contemplate. *I have been eating all my life. Everybody knows how to eat. Anyone looking at my frame, before I became ill with GBS, can observe I am a culinary expert. I do not need a therapist to teach me how to eat,* I surmise.

How wrong I am!

I am excited. It will be the first real food entering my mouth in six months. Lorraine comes into my room, not with a filet mignon as I imagine, but with a small container of butterscotch pudding. If I were any more stupid I would have to be watered. My ignorance of my condition is obvious and evident. My thought process is slow to grasp the reality of damage done by GBS.

The hospital bed is cranked up, placing me in a sitting position. Lorraine is accompanied by two other technicians. She carefully instructs me on what will occur. Her main concern is that the pudding goes into my stomach, not my lungs. With their highly technical machine, her assistants are going to be certain the food has not entered my lungs. There is real danger of aspiration.

Lorraine carefully places less then half a teaspoon of butterscotch pudding in my mouth. It is delicious. To me it tastes almost like filet mignon! She instructs me to swallow slowly. I do. It is luscious to my throbbing taste buds. Butterscotch pudding has never been on my menu. To be truthful, I do not normally enjoy it. Still the taste is scrumptious. I am thinking, *I can begin to eat again, even if it is soft food.*

Carefully I swallow the half teaspoon of pudding. It descends, taking the wrong route. I began to aspirate. It is in my lungs, not my stomach!

This ends food-swallowing attempt number one. Lorraine explains my experience is common. With a sweet sympathetic smile she says, "Do not be discouraged. We will try again tomorrow."

With those words she picks up the pudding and departs. I thank her, but want to say, "Please leave the pudding. Just let me taste it and spit it out." Not a good idea, I cannot spit. The left side of my face is still afflicted, like the rest of my body, with paralysis. Later when trying to use a straw, water dribbles down the left side of my cheek.

I fail the eating test. Better to try and fail than to not try at all. The trouble with doing something right the first time is that nobody appreciates how difficult it was. Relearning to swallow will be challenging.

It has not yet occurred to me that I am going to have to relearn every stored physical memory pattern. The human body has a wonderful system of storing routine physical patterns, called engrams. Physical functions we do repeatedly are memorized by our nerves and muscles, so we do not have to concentrate when we perform routine functions. We simply do them. For example, we do not mentally figure out how to pick up a glass, tie a shoe, or open a door. We just do it. Our engram system has this memorized, filed, and stored.

My engram system has been erased through GBS. As I slowly regain my strength and motor skills, I must relearn how to hold a fork, write, tie a shoelace, and even hold a glass. The simplest physical skill must be thought out mentally before being executed. For example, before I attempt to pick up a glass, I must mentally think through the process step-by-step. Before this pattern becomes automatic, the function needs to be executed several hundred times.

True to her word Lorraine returns the next day for lesson number two in eating, or more specifically, swallowing. The first time I aspired. The pudding I swallowed went into my lung. Now she will attempt again to teach me how to get food from mouth to stomach, not mouth to lung.

Instead of being excited, I am apprehensive. Failure the day before has discouraged me. In fact I am slightly afraid to try a second time. Since I cannot yet cough, I can choke while trying to eat.

Lorraine again gives me a very small teaspoon of pudding. Concentrating with all my ability, I cautiously swallow. Eureka! Success! The food slides down the correct tube. Everyone is excited, but not as exhilarated as I.

The technician who accompanies Lorraine has some sort of monitoring device. The medical gadgetry confirms the pudding is where it is supposed to be. If I am careful, I can swallow. Lorraine feeds me half the remaining pudding. This is a positive day on the ledger of progress. Though still paralyzed, I can now swallow food. *Soon*, I think, *I can get rid of the feeding tube, that is surgically inserted into my stomach. My diet will be more than just Ensure!*

For a week now, I have been swallowing pudding. It is time to graduate to solid food. A miniature piece of steak is placed in front of me. The speech therapist cuts a small piece of steak and places it in my mouth. For the first time in six months, I chew. The taste is beyond description. Delicious does not do justice to what my taste buds are experiencing.

After chewing five or six times I stop. My jaws are exhausted; I have not used these muscles for six months. They are so weak I can chew no longer. Atrophy has robbed my jaw strength.

Here comes another formidable task. Strength in my jaw must be rebuilt. Presently this is about the only muscle group I can use. They, however, are so weak that I cannot adequately chew even one sliver of steak! Rehabilitation promises to be the challenge of a lifetime.

The following day another therapist feeds me lunch. The menu is baby-food carrots, mashed potatoes, and beef. For dessert I am given Jell-O. Normally, I would not eat Jell-O. I do not eat anything more nervous than I!

The problem is my stomach has shrunk; I can eat very little. The therapist orders the nurses to cut down on the stomach-tube feeding, so I can eat more. The goal is more food through my mouth, and less with the feeding tube. This proves to be a good idea.

The following day in therapy, placed on the gym mat, I am able to sit upright. The nurses appear shocked, when I scoot my arms forward and back. For the first time I am able to rotate my hips. With the nerve return, I am slowly gaining strength.

It is still two steps forward and one back. Dr. Douglas tells Bess I am on a plateau and will need to get much stronger before moving to the rehabilitation hospital. Dr. Klepper observes both my lungs are still collapsing and soft. To cap off my day, the respiration therapist pumps saline into my breathing tube to make me cough several times. It is just another unpleasant experience. Before I can be free of the respirator, I must be able to cough.

Food is delivered to my room the next day. I cannot eat because no one comes to feed me. Feeding can only be done by the speech therapist. She is nowhere to be found. Apparently this distresses me. By 7:45 p.m. my blood pressure is 215 over 122. My pulse shoots up to 160. By 8:30 p.m. nurses are giving me Procardia and Ativan. This does not help my temperament. My weak body can still recognize unusual trouble.

Dr. Klepper is called by the nurses. The good doctor responds and is soon by my bedside. Immediately he observes that the breathing cuff of the respirator is too deflated. This causes an air loss around it. The result is I am not getting enough oxygen. I am so anxious, my tongue has turned purple. The nurse informs Bess that the milk I was given at lunch causes my secretion to be worse.

The doctor prepares to give me morphine to alleviate my stress and anxiety. Bess requests they hold the morphine for the present. Eventually, my blood pressure decreases to 147 and I fall asleep. This episode reminds me I am not well, though there are many improvements.

It is September 30, my fifth month in the NCC unit, and I am still in isolation. Secretion into my lungs is heavy. Breathing is labored. My color is pale. X-rays are taken revealing I have pneumonia again. The doctor prescribes Cipro, and puts me back on the respirator.

Nursing care is minimal, which frustrates Bess. My paralyzed body is supposed to be turned every four hours. The day passes, and I have not been turned once. Meanwhile, I have become unresponsive. Long experience has taught me, many senior citizens do not die from the illness that brings them to the hospital. Many die from pneumonia.

This will be the worse night I have experienced in the hospital. My pneumonia intensifies. Secretions in my lungs bring labored breathing. I have wanted to die, wanted to live, dedicated myself to getting well, lived five months in NCC on a respirator, had numerous illnesses from GBS, and now I do not believe I will live through the night. The pneumonia, secretions, and labored breathing are a deadly trio.

Compounding my problem is the cold-hard reality that I am a quadriplegic. My strength is zero. I am totally helpless. This is the lowest point in my hospital experience. After making steady progress at a snail's pace, I face my darkest night physically and psychologically.

God has a way of sending special people in great hours of crisis. This night He sends Levi to keep me alive. Levi is a middle-aged gentleman. His receding hairline is complemented by a warm smile that causes his face to glow. Providentially he is assigned to be my respiratory therapist.

Reading my chart, observing me struggle to breathe, and perceiving my frailty, he is intensely concerned about my condition. Levi softly utters that he knows I am critically sick and very uncomfortable. He assures me he will remain by my bedside all night. Sensing my stress, he speaks gently and slowly, almost in a whisper. Thoughtfully, he reveals he has one other patient he will need to help. He utters, "When I leave you it will be for only a few minutes. I will be back with you as soon as possible." His calm spirit is reassuring.

Because of my pneumonia, secretions are increasing. Levi explains he will need to often suction the phlegm from my lungs. He apologizes for the necessity of suctioning me so frequently. The remainder of the night,

Levi and I fight for my life. It seems he is slipping a tube into my trachea opening, suctioning me every five minutes. Sleep is illusive. I am uncomfortable, uneasy, miserable, and distressed. Nevertheless, Levi continues the suctioning throughout the night. Just before dawn, from sheer exhaustion, I fall asleep.

Without Levi's constant care, I would not have lived through the night. The pneumonia would surely have killed me.

After such a difficult night, I awaken with a high fever. My body is aching. Two new antibiotics are given. My body is cold. After being awake most of the night, I am exhausted and unresponsive. The day is spent on the respirator.

Dr. Bissett, who specializes in infectious diseases, examines me to ascertain if a new disease is my problem. After a thorough examination of my charts and body, he determines my medication should be more closely monitored. There is no infectious disease. It is a catch twenty-two since antibiotics are necessary for infections, but the medication causes weaknesses that allow Cdiff. to grow.

I am too sick to go to the gym for rehab. This does not cause me to shed any tears. Going to the gym is a pain. The nurses get me partially dressed, then I am picked up by two attendants and dropped (placed) in a wheelchair too small for my frame. A portable respirator accompanies me. Being in diapers and having a catheter pose special additional problems. Finally, my experience is, when we get to the gym, little is accomplished. The therapists are so concerned about my respirator, catheter, and helplessness, they can do little that is productive.

To my regret, I have seldom exercised as I should. It is a well-known fact that for every minute you exercise, you add a minute to your life. The real advantage of exercising every day is that you die healthier. When I did exercise, it was early in the morning, before my brain figured out what I was doing.

The fourth day of my pneumonia is October 3. My wife is having a really bad day. I am joining her. She is confronted with three new challenges.

Challenge number one: The doctors are being hassled by my insurance carrier. A family member reports to Bess my hospital bill has reached $570,000 and that I should get to a rehabilitation hospital as soon as possible. Previously Bess learned my insurance limit on GBS is one-million dollars. It seems the insurance money will be exhausted before I am well—if I get well. It appears I will need to be placed in a nursing home rather than here in NCC at Seton Hospital. This is demoralizing to Bess and painful to me.

The antidote for fear and worry is faith and truth. Bess calls our health insurance company, PruCare, and inquires about the amount of insurance used. PruCare reports they have paid $259,000 to the hospital. Additionally, there are professional fees for our many doctors. Seton Hospital had indeed billed $570,000, but discounted the bill almost 50 percent. Beyond that the insurance company tells Bess, at the current rate, I could remain in the hospital another 136 days! Things are better than we thought.

There is a cliche often quoted by those of us who are pastors, "Fear knocked at the door. Faith answered. No one was there."

Challenge number two: Dr. Douglas tells Bess I am on a plateau and have made no progress the last ten days. (Remember, he definitely is not an optimist.) He does not see me going to the rehabilitation hospital anytime soon. My color is not good, and my spirits are down. Bess writes in her notes, **"Bad Day!"** It is.

Just three days later my pneumatologist, Dr. Mazza, informs us I do not need the respirator anymore, and will be out of intermediate care in a week. He thinks that very soon I can be transferred to a rehabilitation hospital!

Challenge number three: Lorraine Stewart, my speech therapist, informs us they will perform the barium test this afternoon. This will reveal if I am aspirating food, thus causing lung problems. Tests show some leakage when I swallow. Feeding by mouth has been put on hold.

After thirteen days I take the barium test and pass. Moreover, in the interim I learn to cough. Being able to cough gives me the ability to rid myself of any food that slips into my lungs. *Soon, very soon, I can be free of the respirator.*

Maybe, just maybe, Murphy's Law isn't a *law* after all. Perhaps it is just the misconception of a frustrated pessimist.

In three days my temperature is normal. The x-rays are clear. My pneumonia has been eradicated. Dr. Mazza plans to move me from the Neurological Critical Care Unit to the fourth floor of the hospital next week, if all goes well. If I can tolerate a private room for a few days, I can then be transferred to a rehabilitation hospital. Additionally, I no longer need the respirator. They may use it at night just to conserve my strength. Dr. Mazza again assures my wife I will recover!

To top off the day, Fred Akers visits me. For ten years Fred was head football coach at the University of Texas. The presence of Coach Akers in my hospital room lifts my spirits. He and Diane, his lovely wife, are precious friends. Fred visits for a time and presents to me an autographed hat with the inscription "Faithful Coach."

On October 7, I am on the collar all day. Being free of the respirator is a positive sign. Additionally, I have regained my ability to cough. All of this is good, but I am nervous about leaving NCC. The realization I will be without a respirator near at hand gives me more anxiety. That machine has kept me alive six months! I have become dependent. This phobia will haunt me as I go to the rehabilitation hospital.

I am also concerned nurses will not be just outside my door monitoring my life-support system. Bess understands my fears and promises to stay with me the first few nights in intermediate care. What a wife! I promise to take her on a trip as soon as I am able.

On day 188 in the hospital, I am telling elephant jokes: Do you know why they don't let elephants on the beach? ... They wear their trunks too low.

Know why everyone tries to hire elephants? ... They work for peanuts.

Know how you can tell if you have an elephant in the bathtub with you? ... You can smell the peanuts on his breath.

Preparations are made to move me from NCC in three days. I do not think the jokes are that bad! Doctors Douglas and Weingarten appear to be thrilled with my progress. It has been so slow. Now it appears to be accelerating.

Bess informs me the doctors are amazed to see my condition improve so dramatically.

I am placed on a much smaller vent at night. My breathing parameters are finally 1,000 and holding. My fingers are moving very slightly on both hands.

Christopher Columbus discovered America on October 12, 1492, an historic occasion. On October 12, I move out of critical care and into Seton Hospital, room 409! My respirator is removed. The heart monitor is disconnected. No longer do I have an oxymeter on my finger. There is a large window in my new room. I can see outside. The room is quiet. Bess spends the night with me for the first time in 192 days. We sleep with the lights off, a new experience.

My progress indicates we need the services of a doctor who specializes in rehabilitation. A nurse tells Bess about Dr. Charlotte Smith, a physiatrist, who is an expert in this unique field of medicine. "Contact her," is the nurse's suggestion. After conferring with two of the doctors treating me, Bess phones Dr. Smith.

Promptly Dr. Smith returns Bess' call. My wife explains I have Guillain-Barrè Syndrome and will soon be released to a rehabilitation hospital. Bess concludes by asking, "Will you take my husband as a patient?"

Sympathetically Dr. Smith responds, "I am not taking any new patients. I regret I will be unable to help your husband." She also informs Bess that St. David's Rehabilitation Hospital is full. I will need to find another rehab hospital.

Bess thanks Dr. Smith and asks if she would suggest another doctor who might help. After hesitating for a moment, Dr. Smith inquires, "Is your husband Dr. Ralph Smith, pastor of Hyde Park Baptist Church?"

"Yes."

"Then I will be your husband's doctor. Moreover, I will reserve a room for him at St. David's Rehabilitation Hospital." Dr. Smith then relates, "When I was a teenager I had meningitis. I was in Breckenridge Hospital. Though I was not a member of your church, your husband came to the hospital and visited me. He prayed for me when I was very sick. I have not forgotten his visit and prayer for my recovery. I will be happy to be your husband's doctor!"

There is a providence in life that is beyond understanding. Experience has taught me, "All things work together for good to them who love the Lord." Securing Dr. Smith's expertise proved to be a gift from God. She is a genius in rehabilitation!

Dr. Charlotte Smith visits me the next day and indicates that by Monday, I should be able to move to St.

David's Rehabilitation Hospital. They will work to get rid of all tubes, start the assessment on Monday, and begin serious rehab the next week. Furthermore, she informs us, a room has been reserved for me directly across from the nurses station. I am so excited I want to shout!

With my euphoria I am able to tolerate the tilt table for twenty minutes in the afternoon. This machine slowly tilts a patient to a standing position. After being bedridden for an extended time, when standing, patients may experience dizziness, high or low blood pressure, or clamminess.

I have considerable difficulty with this gradual elevation from lying flat, to moving to a standing position. I request the therapist to simply elevate me directly to a standing position without hesitating every few degrees. The hardwood surface on the tilt table is hurting my back. I am confident I can tolerate being upright.

This is not the normal procedure There is considerable discussion.. Finally, the therapist stands me upright.

I am standing!

Yes, they have me strapped in and immobile, but standing nevertheless. For over 190 days I have been flat on my back. Being in a standing posture is refreshing.

After twenty minutes I am back in a reclined posture, exhausted.

The next four days, good men from our church stay in my room throughout the day. At night my wife, or daughter, is with me. My breathing remains strong. Daily I receive passive exercise. It is evident I am gaining strength, and increased lung capacity.

My tenure in Seton Medical Center is rapidly coming to a close. I have survived NCC. After six-and-one-half months, I am finally able to be transferred to a rehabilitation hospital. I surmise: *Nothing can be more painful and difficult than what I have endured.*

How wrong I am!

# The Rehabilitation Hospital

October 17, 1995, is an historic day in my recovery process. After 196 days I am well enough to be transferred to a rehabilitation hospital. My heart is overflowing with happiness because my body is restoring itself, overcoming the GBS.

I am happy that I am going to St. David's Rehabilitation Hospital. Many other emotions are going through me. Joy is the primary mood of my mind. But apprehension and fear are running a close second. I have improved enough to be out of NCC, moved to a private room, and now a rehab hospital. I am, however, a weak quadriplegic unable to do anything for myself. Running through my mind is the question: *How can I do rehabilitation when I can't move?*

Two EMS attendants skillfully place me on a gurney, remove me from my Seton Hospital room, and put me in an ambulance. After a short ride we arrive at Saint David's Rehabilitation Hospital. The attendants remove me from the ambulance, wheel me through the hall, into an elevator, and deliver me to my new hospital home.

Nurses give me a sense of security. They have been keeping me alive for half a year. I have grown accustomed to their constant care. Two nurses and two attendants are at the elevator to greet the paramedics and me, when we arrive on the third floor. As they lead us into room 300, they appear happy, cheerful, and enthusiastic. Ann, the charge nurse, introduces me to David, Leah, and two other attendants. For some reason, I cannot understand, they refer to me as a celebrity. Though I do not see myself as a celebrity, the dignitary treatment makes the day perfect.

Words are inadequate to describe my pleasure with room 300, my new home. It is a large, bright room bathed in sunlight shining through three windows. From these windows I can see the upper deck of Interstate 35 that runs through the heart of Austin. Directly across from room 300 is the nurses' station, giving me additional assurance.

Immediately I observe there is a respirator in the room. This is reassuring, since I have depended on one to keep me breathing for six months. Today is Monday and I have been fully off the respirator since Friday, only three days. I am tense and apprehensive regarding my breathing. Having the respirator available is encouraging.

Nurses are highly intelligent in medical matters, and aware of the patient's psyche. The nurses apparently realize how dependent on the respirator I have been, and evidently still am. Thus there is a respirator in my room. What I do not realize—it is disconnected! It is here purely for psychological reasons. It is good I do not know it is inoperative. My comfort level would be zero.

Entering the rehab hospital, I presume my stay will be brief. My misguided thinking is: *I will be here six weeks or less. It will not be long before I am back home.* This unfounded optimism adds to my cheerful mood. Truth is, room 300 Saint David's Rehabilitation Hospital will be my home for six months, not six weeks.

I am happy because of what I do not know. Had I realized the length of time, pain, and frustration I am about to endure in the rehabilitation process, I might be reluctant to begin. On second thought, my stubborn tenacity is adequate motivation. I intend to do whatever is necessary to recover.

As the days go by, my progress is exceedingly slow, and although I do not appear to be progressing, adjusting to the rehab hospital has been a relatively easy transition. Without exception the nurses, therapists, attendants, and other personnel are polite, courteous, friendly, and helpful. On a grade system, all the St. David's team deserves an A-plus. The night crew does, however, function in a different way.

My nights in St. David's Rehabilitation Hospital are a comedy of errors. Some of the problems are mine, but the night staff deserves their share of credit.

At 7:00 p.m. when the late-shift nurses arrive, Mary, the Charge Nurse, and her LVN assistant introduce themselves to me. Both are smiling, encouraging, and inquire if I need anything.

"Yes, I would appreciate having a respirator in my room." After living on a respirator six months, I have remained troubled since it was removed.

The night nurse points out there is oxygen available in my room located directly above my head. This fails to bring me any assurance. My concern is **there is no respirator in my room!**

Whoever wrote: "Fear is not real" has not experienced *real* fear. The fear may have no reality in fact, but the emotion of fear is undeniable! As I am getting ready to go to sleep, my mind is thinking, *What will I do if I have breathing problems?* My thought process is: *If I develop a breathing problem there is no respirator immediately available. I will die. If I don't die, I will have to again endure the choking/drowning feeling I frequently experienced in NCC, when they suctioned my lungs. My overwhelming trepidation is not without experience.*

To give me assurance, the attendant brings in a special nurse-call apparatus. It is placed on the pillow next to my cheek. By turning my head and pushing with my cheek, I can alert the nurses' station. As yet, I cannot press a button with my finger, but hopefully I can press the cheek pressure pad. With it I can summon a nurse, if I need help.

The problem is, I discover, that calling a nurse and getting a nurse are not the same. Mary boasts that now I have "The First Team" caring for me. She lets me know her crew is "The First Team." Perhaps her boast is to assuage my anxiety. I say to myself, *Relax, they will take care of me.*

Mary's next few sentences shatter my lofty expectations. She, with little subtlety, informs me their floor has the maximum number of patients. They are lacking sufficient help, and consequently, are overworked. Moreover, several patients on third floor require almost constant care. In short, I must understand *not* to call, unless I am standing at eternity's door with the death angel behind me pushing.

*Oh well, that's okay. I have been fed. I am warm and safely tucked in bed. What can I possibly need?*

The urinal!

I have active kidneys and a tiny bladder. Around 2:00 a.m. I awaken with an urgent need to urinate. Later the nurses will teach me to say, "I need to pee." For some reason, unknown to me, they like that better. It does get to the point. Anyway, I need to exude some liquid from my bladder PDQ! Having recently discarded the catheter, I am proud to be continent.

With a Herculean effort I am able to slightly turn my head and press my cheek on the nurse-call apparatus. No one responds. Did my cheek pressure activate the button? With no response I cannot be certain I have alerted the nurses. I wait an hour, not really, just five or ten minutes, and press the button again. No response. Pressure builds, and I am desperate. My first night off the catheter is not the time to wet the bed. I do not want the catheter to be reinserted.

In my desperation I call as loudly as I can, "Nurse!"

An adamant voice answers through the speaker system over my bed, "What do you want?" Though the answer is not warm or friendly, it is like a voice from heaven.

"I need a urinal."

Response, "Just a minute."

The minute turns out to be ten. That is okay. I am continent! Incidentally, that in itself is a minor miracle, after being on a catheter six months.

Finally, and not a minute too soon, a huge nurse appears. My bladder is about to explode. My face is getting red. Help is here, at last! I am about to get relief, but not immediately. First, the nurse washes her hands slowly, and thoroughly. That would normally be good. At this moment, however, I am only interested in getting the urinal. Then she puts on her latex gloves. Next she asks, "Where is the urinal?" I am thinking: *How should I know? I can't get out of bed!* After a search she finds the urinal in the bathroom. Pulling back the bedcover, she positions the urinal for me and then turns to leave the room.

"Wait!" I call after her. "Please get me deeper in the urinal. You will need to hold the urinal."

The nurse, who is large enough to play tackle for the Green Bay Packers, looks at me as if I have lost my mind. "It will be fine. I have propped up the urinal. Call me when you are finished. I will be back in ten minutes."

Who am I to argue with a nurse? She would not listen anyway. Advice is something the wise don't need and fools won't accept. Maybe I am different, but it does not take me ten minutes to pee. The urinal starts to tip over. With my arms and hands paralyzed, I can do nothing to prevent it. The urinal falls over and the bed is sopping wet. My legs are drenched in urine. The nurse is nowhere to be found.

True to her word, in ten minutes she returns.

It is unnecessary to tell her the bed and patient are wet. She is frustrated and cannot understand why the urinal spilled. I know the answer, "No one held it." It takes patience and restraint not to say, "I told you so!"

Instead I meekly say, "I am sorry." My theory is always, keep your words soft and sweet, just in case you have to eat them. I do feel sorry for my overworked nurse. She has many patients with various challenges. Apparently, she fails to grasp, I am totally paralyzed.

After a considerable amount of time, another nurse is summoned. By making me wait in a urine-soaked bed, perhaps they are trying to teach me a lesson. Presumably they are occupied elsewhere. They begin to strip the bed one side at a time. Since someone has to roll me on my side to remove the wet linens and put new linens on the bed, a third nurse is called to help. When this has been done on one side, I am rolled to the other side of the bed and the process is repeated. The nurses then bathe my legs and privates.

It is evident the nurses are not exactly happy. Neither am I. The accident could have been prevented. Some nurse needs to hold the urinal steady. This is not going to happen. The whole process consumes an hour, or longer. Had she held the urinal, it would have taken less than two minutes.

All of this episode occurs in the middle of the night. I am grateful I never required much sleep. I refuse to complain about my urine bath. I am not a grouch. A grouch thinks the world is against him----and it usually is. William Shakespeare penned:

*Sweet are the uses of adversity ...*
I remember the discerning words of Samuel Johnson:

*Adversity has been considered the state in which a man most easily becomes acquainted with himself.*

Interestingly enough, this same process is repeated many times. I plead with the nurse to hold the urinal in place. The nurse tells me it is not necessary. She then leaves the room. Her mind is like concrete—permanently set. Upon her return the urinal is tipped over, I am wet, and so is the bed.

Though I do not know it at this time, I will remain in the rehab hospital for six months and two weeks. My experience the first night will often be repeated. The night nurses can't bring themselves to stand by my bed and hold the urinal. Putting myself in the nurses' position, I cannot be too critical of them. If I were a female nurse, I would not want to hold a urinal while a male patient urinates.

Einstein once said: "An idiot is a person who repeats exactly what he has done before, expecting a different outcome." The night nurses keep repeating the same urinal procedure, expecting a different outcome. Maybe they enjoy changing my bed in the middle of the night?

My optimistic mood saves me from being distressed with the process. It eventually becomes entertaining. I realize I am developing a warped sense of humor, but it preserves me from germinating a negative attitude. I am beginning to view the night urination as a comedy routine. Out of every event comes experience and knowledge. I credit the night nurses for sharpening my sense of humor. My six months in NCC has certainly dulled my sense of jocularity. It is hard to laugh with a tracheotomy tube in your throat. These nurses restore my merriment.

For several weeks I have a good chuckle after they leave my room. Having changed the wet bed, they are grumbling and slightly frustrated. I am amused. One benefit of the urinal spill is getting fresh sheets every night there is a spill.

The routine never changes except on weekends. The Saturday and Sunday nurses hold the urinal. I look forward to Saturday and Sunday.

Even with this nightly spilling episode, I admire and appreciate the night crew. They are overwhelmed with duties. There are far fewer nurses at night than during the day. Additionally, the day crew of nurses have therapists assisting. It is more difficult serving on the night crew. All who help me are skilled, attentive, and dedicated to being helpful. They have my love, respect, and admiration.

114

Dr. Smith is thoughtful enough to give Bess a written report of her analysis of my condition. It pointedly summarizes my feeble physical condition.

*EXTREMITY EXAMINATION:* The patient has active motion with approximately 10 degrees range of motion in flexion and extension. There is no active motion to the elbow, wrists, or fingers. The same is noted of the lower extremities. The patient has no active range of motion to the lower extremities. Sensation and proprioception intact, however, throughout all extremities. Trace hip abductors, but no hip flexors or extensors. The patient is quite orthostatic and tolerates only 60 degrees of head of bed up. Heel cords are noted to be quite tight. However, the patient can be brought to neutral. There are no other contractors. It is noted that the patient has marked discomfort and pain throughout any range of motion to the upper and lower extremities.

Diagnosis:
1. Guillain-Barrè Syndrome.
2. Respiratory failure with tracheotomy, stable.
3. Hypertension.
4. Sleep apnea by history.

*TREATMENT PLAN AND GOALS:* Reverend Smith will receive physical therapy, occupational therapy, medical and nursing management to address the problems listed above. The patient *will receive intensive respiratory therapy directed at completing the wean off the ventilator. However, at this admission he has been off the ventilator for two nights and anticipates hopefully not using the ventilator. The patient, when appropriate, will have aquatics therapeutic reaction and spinal cord education will be initiated.*

Unknown to me is the daunting task of my body rebuilding itself. This process defies imagination, or description. I am totally paralyzed. The myelin sheath covering of my nerves needs to be restored. My ligaments have tightened and must be stretched before I can become functional. Atrophied muscles will need to be awakened and rebuilt. Function needs to be restored to my arms, hands, and fingers. At this moment I am more helpless than a newborn baby—an infant moves, I can't.

Meeting these challenges, I must next relearn how to do all physical functions. My engram system has been erased. All learned physical memory patterns will have to be relearned. For a brief moment I am so euphoric over arriving in the rehab hospital, I am contemplating none of these challenges. Future challenges are not going to ruin this thrilling first day.

My mind is contemplating the improvement I have made. My physical improvement is in two important areas. The first, and most critical, is my breathing. Nerves, muscles, etc. that operate my lungs have rebuilt, and are functioning with frailty. The therapist has weaned me off the respirator. However, the anxiety attacks that harried me in NCC have not disappeared. This phobia regarding my breathing continues to plague me. I am grateful the respiratory therapist will work with me daily to increase my lung capacity.

My ability to swallow food is the second area of improvement. Possibly I would not have been admitted to the rehabilitation hospital if I were still unable to swallow. My chewing ability is extremely weak. It is still mandatory for a speech therapist to feed me. Fortuitously, my stomach has shrunk. Little chewing is necessary because my stomach feeding tube is still in place.

*What will be the outcome of my illness?* In my hours of loneliness I contemplate where this journey will ultimately end. *Will I be in a wheelchair? Will I be bedfast? Will I ever reach a point where I feed and dress myself? How long will it take me to recover, if indeed I do recover? If I end up helpless and bedridden, what nursing home will my wife choose? Can we afford a nursing home? It will be physically impossible for Bess to care for a quadriplegic. What then will we do? Will our finances be adequate?*

There are many questions and few answers. With absolutely zero control over any of these challenges my faith must be strong—in God, family, doctors, nurses, friends, and the future.

One thing is certain. Had I known what lay ahead, my mood on day one in rehab would not be joy and happiness! The Rehabilitation Hospital will quickly eliminate anyone without strong resolve. Rehab is a long, hard, difficult, frustrating, tiring, painful process. Therapists request the patient to do exactly what he cannot do. It is a stretch of mind, will, resolve, and body. Progress is slow, measured in minuscule gains.

# No Pain, No Gain

*A*s I awaken on my first full day in the rehabilitation hospital, I am greeted by the charge nurse Ann, and two nurses' aides. It is obvious they are anticipating getting me on a schedule. Before they can complete their information session, Dr. Smith enters the room and stands at the foot of my bed. She greets me with a bright smile and cheerful "Good morning."

Dr. Smith was born to be a physiatrist. A physiatrist (pronounced fizz ee at' trist) is a physician specializing in physical medicine and rehabilitation. Physiatrists treat a wide range of problems from sore shoulders to spinal cord injuries. Simply put, they attempt to restore function to people, whether it is a spinal cord injury, brain injury, stroke, amputations, multiple sclerosis, or in my case, GBS.

She is the Administrator of Saint David's Rehabilitation Hospital. Additionally, she is nationally recognized as one of the outstanding physiatrists in America. Frequently, she lectures at medical meetings. Conceivably, she could spend all her time giving lectures on her specialty. She is foremost in her field. Later I learn that Dr. Smith is married to skilled surgeon, Dr. Ames Smith, Jr.

Dr. Smith is a very attractive lady with a winsome personality. She has black hair and brown eyes sparkling with intelligence. She is attired in her white doctor's coat. Her approach is direct. "I am going to do everything I can to help you get well."

At Dr. Smith's side is a handsome young man. "This is my associate, Dr. Richard Harris. He will also be helping you." She holds a copy of my daily schedule in her hand and explains the daily agenda. It includes physical therapy (PT), occupational therapy (OT), and respiratory therapy (RT). The schedule is then posted in my room and on the hallway bulletin board.

The agenda is explicit. Goals are set by the doctor, therapist, and patient. Progress is measured, noted, and charted daily and monthly. It involves recovery, recuperation, convalescence, mending, and finally restoration. The process is called *rehabilitation*. It is a slow process. Minuscule gains are recorded and treasured. Impatience must be resisted.

Perseverance is the key to successful recovery. Failure occurs often. This must not discourage my recovery. The calamity in rehab is not to fail, but to fail to try again.

My belief is: *I am not a failure until I give up. Failure does not make me a failure.*

120

\* \* \* \* \*

When Rome ruled the known world, a breathless courier reported to Julius Caesar, "We lost the battle."

Reportedly Caesar responded, "Return to your commander. Tell him Rome does not go to battle, Rome goes to war!"

I am not in a battle. I am in a war fighting GBS. One, two, or two-dozen failures mean nothing.

Herein is the challenge: Rehabilitation seeks to get the patient to do exactly what he cannot do. I agree with Victor Hugo: "People do not lack strength; they lack will." My will is about to be tested with Dr. Charlotte Smith's schedule of my rehabilitation.

<u>Ralph Smith's Daily Schedule:</u>

7:30 a.m.   -   Respiratory Therapy with Dave or Levi
9:00 a.m.   -   Speech (Feeding)
9:30 a.m.   -   Rest
10:00 a.m. -   Physical Therapy with Rob
10:30 a.m. -   Therapeutic Recreation with Becky
11:00 a.m. -   Respiratory Therapy
11:30 a.m. -   Psychiatry with Colleen (Wednesday)
Noon         -   Lunch
Rest
1:00 p.m.   -   Pool with Jeff or Greg

2::30 p.m. -   Occupational Therapy with Katie

3:00 p.m. -   Continue Physical and Occupational Therapy
(Rob & Katie)

5 - 9 p.m. -   Dinner and Visitors allowed


Hearing the schedule I feel relieved. There are two rest breaks each day. It appears to be an easy, relaxed program. What I fail to realize is that this is the proposed schedule. It is where I begin, and is subject to change as I progress.

Change, however, occurs within a week or so; I develop Cdiff. again. I am anticipating being in the pool daily. Water therapy is one of the better tools in rehabilitation. With diarrhea I cannot use the pool. This is my first of many disappointments in the rehab process.

I accept the fact that some days I am the pigeon and some days the statue.

My next frustration is in my blood count. It is not good. Consequently, Dr. Helmer has the lab draw blood most mornings. I donate, not voluntarily, at 6:00 a.m. each morning, Monday through Friday. Fortunately, the lab technician who extracts my blood is experienced. Never does he miss my vein, causing a second stick. His skill amazes me. The blood extraction is quickly accomplished.

The respiratory therapist arrives at 7:30 a.m. He employs several instruments to expand my lung capacity. Since my breathing remains very shallow, I continue to need daily respiratory therapy. These exercises in deep breathing are exhausting.

Fortunately, I have three, primary, young aggressive therapists: Rob, Katie, and Becky. They revise the schedule we will follow, until I am able to enter into pool therapy. Thus the modified schedule is:

| | | |
|---|---|---|
| 7:30 a.m. | - | Respiratory Therapy |
| 9-10 a.m. | - | Occupational Therapy |
| 10-11 a.m. | - | Gym |
| 11-12 a.m. | - | Physical Therapy |
| Noon | - | Lunch |
| 1:00 p.m. | - | Classes on Rehab and Respiratory Therapy |
| 2:00 p.m. | - | Gym |
| 3:00 p.m. | - | Occupational Therapy |
| 4:00 p.m. | - | Physical Therapy |

During the ensuing months I learn to appreciate and admire Dr. Smith. Regardless of the challenge of my paralysis, she always seems to know exactly what to do. If plan "A" does not work, she has plan "B." Undiscouraged by every failure I have, she patiently works with me through the therapists to restore my feeble health.

I do not remember anything but positive encouragement from Doctors Smith or Harris. This does not mean they do not talk frankly and candidly with me regarding progress or deficiency. Additionally, they demand my therapists work me strenuously every day. At times I feel they push me too hard. I think I am the only patient in the hospital who is given physical therapy on Saturday and, occasionally, Sunday.

Beyond visiting in my room each morning, Dr. Smith often is in the gym or at the swimming pool observing my progress and instructing the therapists. Dr. Smith is not only professional, but obviously takes a personal interest in my progress. Dr. Harris is equally dedicated to my healing. I am most fortunate to have their discerning and skillful direction.

One occurrence made me extremely happy during my first week at St. David's Rehabilitation Hospital. My wife and daughter informed me they were going to take a short four-day vacation. They mentioned that they had planned on taking the vacation as soon as they were sure that I had progressed to the point where I could be by myself overnight. With the move to the rehab hospital, and their confidence in Dr. Smith, it seemed like the perfect opportunity for them to go.

How can their absence from Austin bring me satisfaction? I love my family more than life. My wife has been at the hospital daily, often staying through the night. I sense she is exhausted. It greatly pleases me that she and my daughter Diane are taking a few days of vacation. They need it!

There are few things in life more tiring than visiting a relative or friend in the hospital. Having been a pastor nearly fifty years, visiting people in hospitals three to five days a week, I am a self-appointed expert on hospital visitation. It is challenging, tiring, time-consuming, and often depressing.

For example, just getting to the hospital is a test of patience. Driving time can be fifteen to thirty minutes. If visiting a hospital in Austin, you park in the hospital garage. Finding a place to park in the garage requires patience, and is expensive. Often the only parking place is on, or near, the top floor. My humble, but accurate, observation is that the marked-off spaces are designed for subcompact automobiles. After parking (if fortunate enough to find a space) the visitor will now get his or her exercise for the day.

Put on your hiking boots because you will walk several street blocks to the hospitality desk to locate the patient's room number. Now saunter to the elevator, and finally to the patient's room. Thoughtful visitors stop at the nurses' desk, to inquire if it is permissible to visit the patient. Often the visitor is requested to wait.

When entering the patient's room all manner of challenges present themselves. Often the doctor or nurse is with the patient. The patient may be sleeping. Perhaps others are visiting, and it is necessary to wait until they depart. From time to time the patient is out of the room undergoing tests or x-rays. Visiting hours in NCC are specific and limited. It requires planning to be at the NCC Unit the exact hour visitation is permitted.

I have visited many patients in isolation. Before entering the room, it was necessary to put on gown, gloves, and a surgical mask. This is done to protect the patient, visitor, and others. Upon leaving, the first stop is to thoroughly soap and scrub one's hands.

I perceive my wife and daughter are weary. They have daily gone through this tiring and time-consuming process to visit me in the hospital. Getting out of town for a few days will renew their energy. It makes me happy to see them get some needed rest and recreation.

I am also pleased to know I have progressed enough for them to feel comfortable leaving town. Actually, their absence gives me a feeling of independence. That is humorous. I am totally reliant on others. If you cannot move an arm or leg, you are dependent. At least my family knows I have reached the point that they do not have to constantly be with me. This is a recovery milestone and a confidence builder for me!

Another happy occurrence that takes place on my first day at the rehab hospital happens after Doctors Smith and Harris leave the room. The charge nurse and her aides return. All are bright, cheerful, and joking. They inform me that Frederick is assigned to help me. As this announcement is made, the group chuckles; I detect inside humor, not understood by me. I imagine they have assigned me an incompetent aide. Had I known Frederick, as I do now, I would have profusely thanked the charge nurse.

Frederick is slightly over six-feet tall. He has piercings, ocean-blue eyes, and long dishwater-blond hair. His eyes sparkle with intelligence and mischief. He is warm, personal, and always ready and willing to help me, or anyone who needs assistance. Always walking on tiptoes, he bounces as he moves from room to room. He possesses a happy servant spirit. Perhaps he acquired it from his father, who is a devout Lutheran pastor. Were I starting a new business, Frederick is the first person I would try to employ.

No patient could have a more caring and efficient nurse than Frederick. He challenges me to improve and comforts me when I am down. He appears up to any challenge. Caring for me will be a formidable task!

Since it is my first full day in rehab, Frederick offers to let me stay in bed and eat my breakfast. Breakfast is delivered and my bed elevated to a sitting position. Frederick proceeds to feed me flawlessly. Hitherto, only the speech therapist has fed me. Apparently, Frederick is trained in this art. The only difficulty we encounter is that I prefer small bites. Frederick, apparently, eats his food in giant chunks. Having made the adjustment to small-bite sizes, he feeds me breakfast. It is a long, slow process.

Following breakfast a portable potty is brought from the bathroom and placed in the center of my room. The staff intends to get my bowel movement (BM) on a regular schedule. This will prove interesting—I was last potty trained when I was a baby. Having been in diapers these six months, it will be a pleasure to sit on a portable potty.

With his strong arms, Frederick lifts me off the bed, and gently places me on the portable potty. Like a king on his throne, watching "Good Morning, America," I have a BM. Frederick stands near me to make sure I do not fall off my throne. I am unstable sitting upright without support.

This is Potty Training 101.

Curiosity is one trait we all possess. My room is directly across from and nearest to the third-floor nurses station. Consequently, three nurses appear in the room to check on my progress. I am wondering what they can do to help. The old adage is accurate: The only time the world beats a path to my door is when I am on the potty.

For several weeks this will become my daily ritual. It works! Getting on a regular BM schedule becomes my first step of progress in the rehab hospital. This may seem humorous and inconsequential, but it is most important. For nearly seven months I have been wearing diapers. Shortly this will end. Once again, I can feel like an adult. When necessity forces an adult to diapers, dignity is eroded, and potentially destroyed.

Having successfully completed my initial lesson in Potty Training 101, Frederick cleans me. Wearing diapers is demeaning. Having Frederick clean my backside is infinitely more humiliating. Completing this menial task, Frederick leaves the room and re-enters pushing a wheelchair.

There are various makes and models of wheelchairs. My specified model is antique. It appears to be a discard from World War I. The back is tall enough to support my shoulders and head. There are supports for my legs and feet. Wheels appear larger than most models. The arms are wide enough to allow my arms to rest on them. It is not portable, but can be reclined. It is much larger than any wheelchair I have ever encountered.

Effortlessly Frederick lifts me from the portable potty and deposits me in my new wheelchair. Doris, a lovely, sensitive LVN from Central Africa, pushes my chair to the wash basin. For the first time in months I stare at my ashen face. I am shocked! I do not realize how grim my features have become. Sensing my shock, the LVN smiles and promises to improve my countenance. She possesses a sweet, gentle spirit.

First she washes my face with warm soapy water. This is very refreshing. Next, she prepares to brush my teeth. Taking my toothbrush she deposits toothpaste on the bristles. With her index finger she spreads the paste over and into the bristles.

"Open your mouth and I will brush your teeth."

"I appreciate your help, but first would you please clean the paste off my toothbrush. Thoroughly wash the brush and put new toothpaste on it. Please do not spread the toothpaste with your finger."

With a smile and a trace of bewilderment Doris responds, "I *always* smear the paste on the bristles, when I brush my teeth."

"I appreciate that. You are, however, going to brush *my* teeth. Please do not spread the toothpaste with your finger."

We both have a good laugh. She then brushes my teeth, a special treat. I do not recall having my teeth brushed in NCC. They were occupied keeping me alive. This dear, sweet lady helps me every weekday morning for the remainder of my hiatus in the rehabilitation hospital. No one could be more caring and gracious.

It has been a busy morning and therapy has not even begun. Three of my therapists, Rob, Katie, and Becky, enter my room informing me it is time to begin therapy. All three are young. It is obvious they are challenged by my condition and are ready to initiate the therapy process. Katie is my occupational therapist. This entails gaining use of my arms and hands. Rob, my physical therapist, will help me to walk and use my body. Becky will work with me in the large gym in strengthening exercises.

We begin. Katie informs me she will lift and transfer me from the hospital bed to my wheelchair. Dubious of her ability to transfer me from my bed, with a chuckle, I ask, "Do you know how much I weigh?"

"I *can* transfer you."

My bed is elevated slightly higher than the wheelchair. Rob sits me on the side of the bed. Katie positions her right arm under my legs, and her left arm around my back. My paralyzed right arm is draped over her shoulder.

She intends to hold me like a baby in her arms, swiftly lifting me to the wheelchair.

Katie is a bright, attractive young lady weighing about 130 pounds. My weight is 198. I perceive she can't

131

transfer me. Still, she is so confident. I reason: *The worst thing that can happen is I will end up on the floor in Katie's lap— That's not so bad! Just keep a sense of humor, Ralph. You are about to end up on the floor.*

Katie counts, "One, two, three ..." and with all her strength she gently lifts me off the bed. In the same motion, she moves me toward the chair. Her knees buckle. We slowly descend to the floor.

She is on the floor. I am in her lap. We are wedged between the wheelchair and bed. Somehow Rob reaches out and softens our descent. Now all three of us are on the floor.

Soon I am situated in the wheelchair. Other than Katie's pride being hurt, no harm is done. They fake a nervous laugh, informing me this incident will initiate an abundance of paperwork. I put on my somber face, informing them, "I have two sons who are lawyers. You will hear from both tomorrow."

Having just met me, they can't discern whether I am joking or serious. Immediately, they apologize, express regret, and appear contrite. After a long moment, I laugh. Their anxiety disappears.

Katie rolls me down the hall to a most interesting area. As we enter, there is a bathtub, commode, and various bathroom fixtures. Further inside is a small area with kitchen cabinets, plastic dishes, glasses, and silverware. We use none of these. Katie's interest is in an oval-shaped plastic container. In it is hot, melted wax.

Katie lifts my right hand and gently places it in the hot wax. She lifts my hand out. It is coated with the wax. This dipping is repeated seven times, until my hand is heavily coated with the wax. Quickly she wraps my hand in saran wrap. She then covers it with a towel. The process is repeated with the left hand.

After ten minutes the towel, Saran wrap, and hot wax are removed. The wax has formed a glove coating over my hands and is easily stripped away.

She returns me to my room for my first encounter with occupational therapy (OT). With her hand covering my fingers, she bends them into a fist. For six months these fingers have been straight. My joints are stiff. Without the hot-wax treatment, I do not believe she could have bent the fingers into a fist. This process is repeated several times on both hands. She bends my wrist a far as possible. Though done slowly and gently, I am experiencing sharp pain.

"Now try to bend your fingers." I try but can't move fingers or wrist. Katie continues to move my hand. She bends each finger. There is little flexibility in my fingers.

Having worked on my hands and wrist, Katie lifts my arm and bends my elbow. I shudder with pain. She can only slightly bend my elbow. The goal is to stretch my elbow ligaments until I can place my hand behind my head. This first day she cannot bend the elbow enough to touch my nose. Bending my elbow, stretching ligaments, brings the most severe pain I have ever experienced.

My arms have lain straight out by my side for six months. Ligaments have tightened. They must be stretched before I can bend my arms to do anything useful. This passive exercise proves to be the most dreaded of my therapeutic exercises. The only comfort I have—it is done first each day. This gets it out of the way, so I do not have to go through the day dreading the stretching of elbow ligaments.

Promptly at 10:00 a.m. Becky appears in my room. She rolls me into the elevator, punches the lower level button, and we are on our way to the basement gymnasium. When we enter the gym, I am impressed with all the equipment available. This appears to be the busiest area in the rehab hospital. The equipment is being used by a room filled with patients. Observing the equipment I ponder, *How can any of it be operated by me?*

Becky rolls my wheelchair against a wheel with hand cranks. Rotating the arms forward and backward activates the turning of the wheel. Again I wonder, *Since I can't hold the rotator arms, how can I use the hand bicycle wheel?*

Ace stretch wrapping is the answer. Becky places my hand on one handle, wraps my fingers around the bar and proceeds to wind the stretch wrapping around my hand. Soon my hand is secured to the turning device. She repeats the process with my other hand, firmly securing it to the second hand-crank

"Now turn the handles," Becky commands. I can't. Whoever used the equipment before, set the wheel to resist making it harder to turn. Becky senses my inability and releases the pressure on the wheel. With Becky's help and great effort, I am able to turn the wheel. The rotation is slow, but the wheel is turning as my arms go round and round. The timer is set for five minutes. *Can I last five minutes?* Somehow I manage.

Next, my wheelchair is placed in front of equipment with ropes attached to weights. Again my hands are laced to the handles. With great effort I am still unable to lift the smallest weights. Becky assists. The weights lift slightly with Becky providing the lifting. Since I am unsuccessful pulling the ropes, we move to the next piece of equipment. It is again weights attached to ropes, attached to my hands. This involves bending the elbow to a forty-five-degree angle and slowly releasing until the rope is slack. Again, my strength is apparently zero. *Am I going to be able to use this well-equipped gymnasium?* I ask myself.

Finally, I am positioned facing out from weights behind me. I am to push down on levers lifting the weights. This proves to be my most successful exercise.

Becky starts with twenty-five pound weights, but soon moves to fifty-pound weights. This equipment involves shoulder strength. Here I appear to be the strongest.

During the ensuing weeks, I learn to appreciate the gym. It is a welcome relief from occupational and physical therapy. They are more strenuous and difficult. Here I slowly rebuild my upper-body strength. Becky is consistently encouraging me. Her attitude is positive and her smile is contagious. She becomes a friend, as well as a therapist.

After Becky is through with me, Rob and Katie take me to the third-floor gym. It is a large room with a minimum of equipment ordinarily found in a gym. In this gym are a set of parallel bars, the only piece of equipment familiar to me. Most of the gym is filled with raised, semi-soft, blue mats. The elevation of the mats appears to be eighteen to twenty-four inches off the floor.

Placing his hands and arms under me, Rob swiftly and gently lifts me from my wheelchair, placing me on the edge of the raised mat. Sitting on the mat, my feet rest on the floor. Bracing me he asks, "Can you sit without falling?"

"I believe I can."

Following these words, Rob releases his grip on my shoulders. My shoulders slump severely, but I sit without assistance. Rob stands immediately in front of me and asks me to bend forward, touching my toes. I lean forward unable to reach my gym shoes. With a considerable struggle and Rob's help, I am able to return to my upright sitting position. This is repeated several times. I quickly grow tired. Rob helps me lean back, lying on the mat with my legs dangling to the floor.

Picking up my legs, Rob turns me and places me in a reclined position. I am allowed to lay on the mat for a brief rest. Following this Rob and Katie move me from the edge of the mat, assuring I will not fall off the pad. They request I roll over. This I am unable to do.

Rob and Katie roll me over on my stomach with my arms outstretched in front of me. Somehow they manage to get me up into a crawling stance. My arms are locked and supporting me. I am unsteady, but do not fall. This pleases both therapists. "Try to crawl," is the next request. Unable to move arms or legs, my response is naught. I am becoming exhausted.

"I can't crawl. ..."

Rob corrects me saying, "You can't crawl *yet*."

This simple statement becomes the lock opener to my rehabilitation. When I fail in doing what is requested I say, "I can't do it." My therapists correct my statement by repeating, "You can't do it *yet*." This *yet* infers it eventually will happen. It is a tremendous statement of faith.

It assumes that sometime in the future, I will be able to do what I just tried and failed to do.

Still in my crawling posture, I plead, "Please help me down."

The response is, "Can you lie down on your own?"

"No, but I think I can roll to the side."

"Do that."

With a thud I slip to my right side.

"That was good," Rob utters. Following this he teaches, "You must learn to crawl before you learn to walk." *How stupid I am! This is exactly what babies do—crawl and then walk.* I am reluctant to face the reality I am starting over in leg and arm functions. All the motor skills I lost need to be restored and relearned.

*I am being potty trained and now I'm learning to crawl. I get to experience a second childhood!*

Rob helps me roll over until I am lying on my back. He gently lifts my leg straight up stretching my muscles. When he gets my leg at about a ten-degree angle, I wince. When my leg reaches twenty degrees I cringe with pain. "What are you doing?"

"Stretching your gluteus maximus."

"I do not believe I can stand the pain."

Rob responds, "We have to do it. Without this stretching you will never walk!"

Taking a deep breath I say, "Okay, but I can't help moaning when the pain is so intense. You do what you must. I may scream. I am not angry with you. It helps me to verbalize my hurt. I won't like it, but keep stretching my gluteus maximus, whatever that is."

Rob daily does a good job of stretching my gluteus, and I do a good job moaning in pain every time he stretches them. I realize some people suffer in silence. They could cut the suffering in half, if they would express the felt pain. Why hold it in if you can let it out? A lifetime of experience has taught me verbalizing pain helps rid me of it. Verbally expressing hurt is therapeutic. It is not a panacea, but it brings healing to body and spirit.

Soon I learn that without humor I cannot cope with the intense pain of my therapy. It is either laugh or cry. At times all I can do is cry. Laughing, however, is more appealing. During the ensuing weeks I tell my therapists every joke I know. This diversion takes my mind off my feeble condition and gives the therapists a chuckle. It takes 43 face muscles to frown and only 15 to smile. I'll smile—it's easier than frowning.

My agenda is summarized in the words *hard work*. The therapists push me as hard as they can. It is exercise, exercise, and more exercise. How can I exercise when I can't move arms or legs? The therapists move my limbs for me. They call it *passive* exercise. To me it is not passive. It is *pain* exertion. My muscles are atrophied. My ligaments have shrunk and tightened. This stretching movement is extremely painful and essential.

I am doing my best, which is not very good. It appears we are making no progress. I begin to wonder, *Why am I enduring this painful therapy?* It is a well-known fact that for every minute you exercise, you add a minute to your life. So if you exercise all your life it will enable you to spend an additional five months in a nursing home at $5,000 per month.

After my first week in the rehab hospital, I know I do not have the resolve, strength, or patience to endure rehab. Consequently, I determine to do the following:

First, I must have a tough mind-set. I do not like what has happened to me. My health is gone. My ministry as a pastor dramatically ended. My wife is physically and mentally exhausted. I do not know the status of our finances, but they must be in shambles.

*Forget that! Be mentally tough!*

Second, I intend to concentrate on the goodness of God. When I awake each morning I say to myself: *This is the day the Lord has made, I will rejoice and be glad in it.* Though not happy, I intend to rejoice—as much as possible. I intend to make these days in the rehab hospital good days. I will depend on humor to help me laugh, not lament at my helplessness. My intent is to get better, not bitter. Humor has a way of softening therapy pain. When the therapists are laughing, I observe they ease up on me.

Third, at night alone, before I fall asleep, I will talk with God. He knows my frailty. I will be defeated by what is around me, if I do not get help from the One who is above me. This illness is bigger than I. It keeps me flat on my back months on end. The only One who can heal me is the Great Physician.

Fourth, I totally rest on the rock-solid truth: *"We know that all things work together for good to those who love the Lord."* My illness is not good. God will, however, use it for my good. He loves me, and with all my heart I love Him! So, if my illness will ultimately bring good, why should I fret?

Excellent therapists are working with me six days a week; still I can barely move a muscle. On reflection, this is not entirely true. After a therapist sits me upright, I can sit slightly slumped, with no one supporting. I cannot get myself into a sitting position. On the gym mat I can slowly and slightly move my legs. This requires strenuous effort. I am able to move my arms while lying in bed but cannot lift them. As Tennessee Ernie Ford used to say, "I am like a frog on the freeway with my hopper broken."

\* \* \* \* \*

Before becoming ill my exercise routine was irregular. It seemed that I needed thirty hours in every day. Foolishly, I neglected regular exercise. One day a friend asked me if I jogged. I responded, "No, but I perform a lot of funerals for people who do."

Bad attitude! However, you never have to wonder if a man is a jogger. He will tell you.

One essential in my recovery process is learning to transfer. This is top priority. I can't do this … yet. Since I can't walk (or even stand) I am moved often from bed to wheelchair, or wheelchair to mat, etc. Each move involves the therapist lifting me from one place to another. Thus, my therapists daily help me learn the skill of transferring.

The transfer process is simple. For me, however, presently it is impossible. A flat, smooth board is wedged under my hip. The board extends from my bed to the wheelchair. I am encouraged to scoot on the board from bed to chair. Problem is: I can't scoot.

Rob takes me to the gym and places me on the elevated mat. I am taught to place my hands on the mat and scoot down the mat. With a mighty exertion I move a few inches. "Good!" Rob says, "Do it again." With strenuous effort, I continue this process until I reach the end of the mat.

Though exhausted, I am proud of myself. "Now scoot back down the mat." This takes longer, but is eventually accomplished. Rob explains this is the technique I am to use transferring from chair to mat, etc. This I know I can do.

With a devilish smile Rob parks my wheelchair next to the mat. He wedges the four-foot flat board under my hip. It spans the gap between mat and wheelchair. "Now use the technique you just learned and move to your wheelchair."

With all the strength I have, plus Rob's help and encouragement, I slide on the transfer board from mat to chair. In the process I am gripped by fear. The board could slip off the mat, or chair, dropping me on the floor.

This assisted transfer is the first of many. The process is used every time I move from one place to another. In refining the technique I learn several helpful tactics. First, the transfer is easier if my leg is covered with pants. Sliding skin on board is rugged. Second, it is much easier sliding down. At times I must slide angled up. This is infinitely more difficult. Third, always be certain the transfer board is solidly resting on both ends. It can move in the transfer and cause a fall. Fourth, keep the transfer board smooth. Powder spread on the board is most helpful.

This is a major step in assisting me to become independent. Even though I do not have the grip or strength to hold or place the board, I can transfer with assistance.

In spite of my slow progress, Dr. Smith becomes even more encouraging. She believes I can recover and convinces me I will recover.

The following day, Dr. Smith's husband, Dr. Ames Smith, comes to my room to remove the feeding tube stomach peg. For weeks it has been my primary source of nurture. I surmise he will need to sedate me. He assures me this can be accomplished with little pain and discomfort. After about forty-five minutes the stomach peg is separated from my body. I experience no pain in the process. How thrilled I am to be liberated from a stomach feeding tube.

This is a happy day in the recuperation process.

# The Pain Is Worth the Gain

Following my grooming each morning, Katie, my occupational therapist, arrives to take me to the dining room. It is a culture shock. In the room are fifteen to twenty people with various rehab challenges. I cannot discern what medical problem each individual has, but most appear downhearted. If misery loves company, I am in the right place. The first day in the dining room I could have won the prize for being the most helpless, yet the happiest.

I am barely able to sit in the wheelchair. A safety strap has been stretched across my waist to prevent my slipping out of the wheelchair. The chair is tilted slightly back. This helps to keep me in the chair. If I slip forward, I do not possess strength enough in my arms to prevent my falling out of the chair. My paralyzed legs are of no assistance.

Katie is assigned to feed me. I surmise, this is her first experience feeding a patient with GBS. It is apparent she is not overly excited about this assignment. Later I learn she has only recently completed her master's degree in therapy. Feeding a GBS patient is perhaps a new experience for her.

In NCC the past six months, I have been fed through a tube. The first feeding tube was in my nose going down my throat and into my stomach. The second was the tube surgically inserted into my stomach, recently removed. Now I can swallow. I have had little experience being fed, and Katie apparently has none feeding a paralyzed patient. She feeds me bacon, eggs, toast, and coffee. Except for the coffee, all my food is room temperature. We have a number of laughs. She is cautious and careful. It takes a long while to complete the meal.

When the meal ends I say to myself, *Ralph, get used to this. This will be the way you will eat for several weeks. Relax, laugh, and enjoy the meal—this is preferable to tube feeding.*

I learn several lessons from my breakfast. Do not expect hot food. The helper wants you to eat faster than you are able. Do not order coffee. Drinking it through a straw robs coffee of its flavor. The individual who feeds me will give me much larger bites than I would normally take. Most people salt their food. Consequently, they automatically salt my food. People like to dabble with a fork, and as a result mix food. I prefer each item of food separated from every other item. Expect to have food on your shirt and in your lap. I wear a towel for a bib. Accidents happen!

Being fed by another is one of the more humbling experiences of life. However, I do get fed!

146

Going to the dining room is rewarding. These are but a few of the valuable treasures collected that enrich my life. Eating becomes a challenge and an adventure. I make a number of new friends. Normally three different nurses, aides, or therapists feed me my three meals. They all do it differently. Patience is developed and strengthened. I discover what it means to be "fed like a baby." Finally, none of the inconveniences are important. After being fed through a tube for six months, the taste of any food is a delicious treat!

I am fortunate to be able to chew, taste, and swallow food. Since I have not tasted food for months, any food tastes like gourmet cooking. One of the truly great gifts of life is the sensation of taste. One reason so many Americans are overweight is because we enjoy the taste of food. When dining with others, I am always the last person to finish my meal. The reason is simple. At a leisurely pace, I enjoy chewing food. Now, after being on feeding tubes, I have a new appreciation for taste.

In retrospect, after my illness, I consider every meal a banquet. Seldom, if ever, do I eat a meal without recalling my six months of tube feeding. Every morsel of food is a gift from Heaven. The privilege of eating can never be fully appreciated until it is taken away and later restored. The months I was on a respirator, I longed to drink a Coke in a large glass of ice. Later I dreamed of a medium-well-done thick hamburger with the works—tomatoes, lettuce, pickles, and mayonnaise. Now this longing is being fulfilled.

What a privilege to be healthy enough to eat, chew, swallow, and assimilate food! I do not take this privilege for granted.

Often at lunch friends come to visit. How grateful I am for their company! I never hesitate to ask the visiting friend to feed me. One precious doctor friend, Steve Yurco, feeds me one or two days each week. Three pastor friends, Bruce McMurray, Mark McClelland, and Jim Abingdon (now deceased), have also been good to drop in at noon and feed me. The dining room attendants are overwhelmed trying to feed third-floor patients. These friends, and others, help the staff by feeding me.

By eating in the dining room I have the opportunity to meet most new patients on the third floor of the rehabilitation hospital. I use the word most because a few patients never, to my knowledge, eat in a dining room. One day an elderly man is wheeled into the dining room. A therapist is pushing the wheelchair, and the man's wife follows. His wheelchair is parked at the table across from where I am being fed.

Trying to be friendly, I speak to the couple. She is cordial. He gives no response, though I know he hears and understands me. It is evident he is the victim of a stroke. Since some stroke patients cannot talk, I am not offended by his lack of response. Striking up a conversation with his wife, I welcome them both to third floor. Making small talk, I offer a word of encouragement.

My therapist continues to feed me. I am still learning how to swallow; therefore, I must concentrate on chewing and swallowing my food. However, I discern by overheard conversation that he does not intend to eat. Both his wife and therapist are having little if any success feeding him. He simply will not open his mouth.

I am uncertain how this attempt to feed the new paralyzed patient ends. When I am taken back to my room, they are still unsuccessfully coaxing him to eat. Their patience with him inspires me. Unfortunately, this process is followed daily, with nearly an identical result. Reluctantly, he eats very little. A Missouri mule could not be more stubborn than this gentleman.

He will not speak. He refuses to eat. Day by day it becomes increasingly apparent that he *can* both talk and eat. He *will* do neither. It is evident, he is angry that he is ill. He had not planned on having a stroke. Who does? Now he is unable to cope with the necessity of rehabilitation.

His anger and frustration are defeating him.

During the next several days his wife and I become better acquainted. She is a charming elderly lady. She is both friendly and worried. Learning I am a pastor, she talks with me about her husband's stroke. They live in a small town sixty miles from the hospital. She and her husband recently celebrated their 50th wedding anniversary. Shortly after the commemoration, his stroke unexpectedly occurs. Following a week in their small local hospital, he is transferred to St. David's Rehabilitation Hospital. She explains he would have come sooner, but the hospital was full with no room for additional patients. She feels fortunate he has finally been admitted as a patient. He does not share her enthusiasm.

She tells me her husband has always been independent and robust. Then she goes on to say that the stroke devastated his spirit. In her words, "He is crushed!" The result is he eats little, refuses to cooperate with hospital staff, and will not participate in treatment.

Perhaps she wants my input because when she sees me in the dining room, I appear optimistic, smiling, and laughing. I am constantly sharing jokes, mostly bad, with staff and patients. Had she heard my screams of pain when therapists are stretching me, she probably would counsel with someone else. I am more paralyzed and helpless than her husband, yet remain optimistic. He, on the other hand, is uncooperative, pessimistic, and unwilling to work with therapists. She requests I encourage her husband. I assure her I will.

150

During the course of the next several weeks I make it a point to sit across from her husband as often as possible. We have much in common. Both of us are paralyzed, near the same age, and must to be fed by another. I cannot get him to talk with me. In due time and reluctantly, he does began to eat, though very little.

He steadfastly refuses to participate in therapy. It has become increasingly obvious he is not going to improve. He is unwilling to try to improve. This good man is drowning in self-pity.

He leaves the hospital before I. Being very interested in the man, I ask a therapist if he improved enough to leave.

"No."

"Then why did he leave?"

The answer is diplomatic, "If he will not participate in treatment, he cannot stay in the hospital."

Whether this is his insurance company's policy or hospital procedure, I am uncertain.

Unsatisfied, I ask his therapist if the man *could* have improved. "Without a doubt" is the answer.

The therapist went on to add that he felt the man might have completely recovered. Citing a number of similar cases, the therapist saw no reason why the man could not walk, and perhaps return to his normal lifestyle.

"Certainly," the therapist added, "at the least he could make slow and steady improvement."

I am crushed. When the patient gives up, the doctors, nurses, and therapists can do nothing. If still alive, the gentleman is now bedfast and/or confined to a wheelchair. His aged wife is caring for him, or he is in a nursing home. His lack of hope and determination not only changed his life, but that of his wife. She became his caregiver. He destined himself to a bed or wheelchair.

There is pain and frustration in therapy. There is infinitely more pain and frustration in refusing to work at rehabilitation. My path out of paralysis will prove to be a painful, hard, grueling journey. However, learning to walk, function normally, drive a car, experience freedom of movement, is worth whatever price one pays. The gain is worth the pain.

One of my substitute therapists believes the phrase, "No pain, no gain." When I am straining, trembling, and crying with pain, that phrase is his method of encouragement. It never encourages me! I appreciate the nurse who tells me she does not believe "No pain, no gain." Perhaps both are right. There are times when "No pain, no gain" is the only approach. On the other side of the coin, some things could just as easily be accomplished with a little less pain.

Abraham Lincoln is reputed to have said: "Most people are about as good as they want to be." It is a self-evident truth that most people who are paralyzed get about as well as they desire and work to get.

There are many who are paralyzed and cannot totally recover. Nearly all can and will improve with undiscouraged dedication, persistent prayer, rugged rehabilitation, and hard work.

A failure is not a person who gets knocked down, or is thrown down by illness. A failure is one who will not attempt to recover, wallowing in anger and self-pity. All one has to do to succeed in rehabilitation is get up one more time than he, or she, is knocked down.

The old gentleman I mentioned is most certainly bedfast, if still alive. His pessimistic outlook prevented him from receiving the help offered. What heartbreak for him, and even more painful a tragedy for his loving wife.

I remind myself often, *Ralph, get up one more time than you are knocked down!*

During my six-month, two-week stay in the rehabilitation hospital, I have the privilege of meeting and eating with a great number of people in the third-floor dining area. Their rehab challenges are varied. Several are adjusting to a new knee or hip. Their stay is brief. Others are elderly and trying to gain strength to return home. This often requires weeks of therapy. Saddest of all are young people who are crippled due to an accident. Most of these will remain in a wheelchair.

# Forward and Backward

*O*ne morning in the rehab hospital I am watching television. Athletes are competing in the Olympics. They are perfect physical specimens, while I am a physical wreck, a quadriplegic. Reflecting on my physical strength, which is zero, I begin to cry. The program upsets me.

Observing my melancholy reaction, Frederick senses my disposition. He softly asks, "Can I help you?"

"No."

As Frederick begins to dress me for the day, he becomes even more sympathetic. His next statement is one I will remember forever. "Ralph, going through what you are enduring is harder than winning an Olympic gold medal. When you walk, you will have accomplished more than they. ..."

Through the excruciating twenty-eight weeks in the rehab hospital, I repeat his words to myself again and again. I doubt if Frederick will ever realize what those words mean to me. An encouraging word from a helper inspires me to keep trying to move an arm, leg, or even twitch a finger. None of which I can do at the moment.

155

Dr. Michael Douglas' prognostication was accurate. I take two steps forward and one backward. That is okay. When I go backward, I remind myself, *You can't fall off the floor.* The day will come when I will stand, walk, and graduate from this great rehabilitation hospital.

Bess enters my room one morning bright and early. She is rested and chipper. "Good morning," she says, planting a kiss on my cheek. Her happiness brings joy to my heart. In many ways my illness has been harder on my wife than on me.

I am shaven. My teeth are brushed. I am propped up in bed with a broad smile on my face. This morning all of my medical reports are positive. Good medical reports are a rare happening.

After greeting my wife, I give a bowel movement report. "Bess, I am finally strong enough to sit on my throne every morning. I am beginning to feel like a human being! When Frederick sits me on the portable potty, I am so excited tears well up in my eyes!"

That appears eccentric but, nevertheless, accurate. Over six months ago nurses put me in adult diapers. Every bowel movement has been dirtiness. At last, some of my self-respect is returning. Very soon diapers will disappear from the orbit of my necessity.

I am smiling.

A second problem is decreasing. Dave, the respiratory therapist, has become a good friend. Three times a day he helps me learn to breathe deeper, enlarging my lung capacity. "Inhale, exhale, breathe deeper, suck as hard as you can on this straw, now harder, try again. ..." is his redundant speech. I need it. After being on the respirator so long, my lung capacity is severely limited. My breathing is shallow, and consequently weak.

This day there is no respirator in or near my room. With a goal of 1,000, my reserve air measures 980. Breathing into and sucking on the minuscule straw is working. This excites my therapist. I am making terrific progress in increased lung capacity.

The third positive report is that my leg and arm strength are good and improving. How they can discern I am stronger is beyond my comprehension. I still cannot move, but if the therapist reports I am stronger, I believe him. My judgment is that in order to be a therapist, one must be a visionary.

The fourth is to me the most significant positive step. The charge nurse carefully removes the urethra catheter. In its place I am wearing a urine rubber. Even with my limited medical knowledge, I know that soon I will be continent.

Wow! What a day! I pause again to laugh at myself. I am extremely happy that I have:

- ➢ Had a normal bowel movement on a portable potty.
- ➢ Breathed without a respirator almost a normal amount of air.
- ➢ Shrugged my shoulders, arms, and legs, though I can't use them.
- ➢ Took a pee through a rubber catheter.
- ➢ And there is no longer a plastic tube shoved into my bladder.

I have traveled a long, dangerous path to arrive at this intermediate station on a journey to wellness. Being exuberant over near-normal breathing and a normal bowel movement indicates the measure of my illness. Breathing without the aid of a machine and urinating minus a catheter are cause for celebration. I am thankful, like the sensible person who wrote: "If you can't be thankful for what you receive, be thankful for what you escape."

My body is clawing, scratching, and fighting its way back to health. It is increasingly evident this path back is going to be drawn out. There is a deep chasm between where I am and where I need to go. David Lloyd George said what I sense: "The most dangerous thing in the world is to try to leap a chasm in two jumps." My body must busy itself in bridge building.

At this juncture all I can do is wait on my body to rebuild. My body is probably working overtime to heal, but it seems to be a very slow pace. Centuries ago Isaiah, the prophet wrote: "They that wait upon the Lord shall renew their strength." This is where I am—waiting, and hopefully renewing my strength.

My nurse reports there is a patient with Cdiff. infection just down the hall. Since it is easily transferred my sputum is tested and x-rays are taken. By afternoon my temperature is 101.5 degrees. My face is flushed and my eyes are matted. I have a tight chest. Later in the afternoon my breathing is shallow. I develop diarrhea. The Cdiff. has moved from down the hall to Room 300.

The following day I am placed in isolation. Tests reveal I have Cdiff. and a bladder infection. Dr. Bissett believes my tests are faulty and perhaps I do not have Cdiff. Unfortunately, the tests do indicate Cdiff. Additionally, I develop an eye infection. Dr. Rock, my ophthalmologist, medicates my eyes. I am given Amoxicillin.

Having taken giant strides forward, I once again step backward.

From past experience I know the Cdiff. lasts ten to fourteen days. Somehow I need to rise above this Cdiff. It can delay my therapy and recovery by an additional two weeks. One of the great psychological discoveries of this century is that thoughts control actions. Positive thoughts virtually always produce positive results. My mind affects my moods. My thinking determines my feeling. I can't control the fact I am sick. I can control what I think about my condition, which will control how I feel.

All medical supplies in my room are dumped into the trash. The room is thoroughly cleaned with a strong disinfectant. All of my clothes are laundered. Nurses, attendants, and family entering my room are required to wear caps, gowns, and gloves. I am given very little therapy. Time is standing still.

This affords me an opportunity to consider my future plans. For a number of months I have pondered when to resign as pastor of Hyde Park Baptist Church. When I first became ill, I believed my recovery would be a few short weeks. Over six months have elapsed. I am deeply concerned about the church. The congregation needs a pastor who is physically fit.

Following a long discussion with my wife, I determine to retire effective January 1. After that date I will receive no compensation. I will request the church make it official on March 19, my sixty-fifth birthday. My long-term plan has always been to retire from the pastor's office at sixty-five. I did not, however, intend to retire in this fashion.

My hope is that I will be strong enough by March to preach one last sermon expressing my love for the congregation. Being a shell of my former self, I no longer feel capable of being a pastor. Through the goodness of God, I have been the pastor of Hyde Park Baptist Church over thirty-five years. The congregation has shown loving patience during my illness.

The following day, October 25, starts well. I enjoy a good night's sleep and eat a hearty breakfast and lunch. My lungs, however, need suctioning during the night. The following day, Dr. Utsett informs me I still have the bladder infection. My diarrhea goes from bad to worse. In one hour I have four bowel movements. With all I have endured, (Cdiff., diarrhea, high fever) my bladder infection appears inconsequential.

Ever so slowly, I am rising above the vicissitudes challenging my recovery. I know I am recovering, even with Cdiff. attacking me and the bladder infection causing high fever.

Sick or well, rehabilitation goes on in this hospital. Thus the therapists, Rob and Katie, roll me to the gym in the antiquated high-back wheelchair assigned to me. We go through sitting, stretching, rolling, and bending. Therapy is extremely difficult. With my fever it is even more arduous.

When this difficult day ends, I am informed I will be given a bath. This announcement surprises me. How can I be given a bath? With a wide-open trachea hole in my throat, the incision from the feeding tube, and my fever 101, how can I be bathed?

One of the disadvantages of being totally paralyzed is that I have not had a real bath in six months. This is not to say the nurses have not bathed me. While in NCC the nurses bathed me daily. Taking a wash rag and hospital soap, a nurse scrubs my front side as I lay flat on my back. After doing the best she can to get me clean, two nurses turn me on my side to finish the job. More often than not, however, they do not turn me on my side because of the trachea in my throat, monitors, and tubes attached to my body.

Why wash my backside? I am wearing a diaper. Every time they change my diaper they scrub my backside. Indeed, I am getting a mini bath every time I defecate. But I have not been in a shower or bathtub for over six months.

I am thrilled beyond description when the charge nurse announces they are going to give me a bath. Being of a thoughtful disposition, I wonder, *How are you going to give me a bath?* I am still totally paralyzed. I cannot conceive of any way the nurses can give me a bath. So naturally, I ask, "How are you going to give me a bath?"

"In the Blue Canoe."

"What is the Blue Canoe?" I inquire.

"You will see."

After lunch Frederick and a *female* attendant wheel a gurney into my room. On top of the gurney is a six-foot blue plastic *boat*. The sides are one or two inches high. The end is open. It is jokingly referred to as the Blue Canoe. This is to be my bathtub for the next several months.

The gurney is rolled parallel to my hospital bed, which is elevated to its greatest height. Two additional nurses enter my room. After being rolled on my side, a sheet is placed snug against me. Then I am rolled over the sheet to my other side. The sheet is pulled under me. The nurses position themselves at my head, side, and feet. On the count of three, gripping the sheet, they *almost* hoist me from bed into the Blue Canoe.

I land half-in and half-out of the canoe. With a second attempt, the four nurses succeed in placing me into the Blue Canoe. Now I am lying naked inside the plastic blue receptacle. I imagine this is what a corpse feels like before being embalmed, if it could feel. Not being dead, but stark-naked, I am embarrassed. A thoughtful nurse covers me with a sheet and we are on the way to my first shower in nearly seven months.

Frederick, my assigned nurse during the day, is a practical joker. He keeps himself amused doing his job. He pushes the gurney down the hospital hall with enthusiasm and too much speed. It is propelled toward the nurses standing in the hall. After dodging, they laugh. Apparently they are used to his antics. It is anything but comical to the passenger—me! Fear has replaced my embarrassment.

My mind is conjuring up a host of possibilities, none of which are good. *What if the Blue Canoe falls off the gurney? What if we hit a wall? What if the sheet covering me flies over my head? Under the sheet I am wearing only my birthday suit.* People in the hall are frantically dodging our gurney. Two of them barely escape Frederick's seemingly reckless steering! I can picture a nurse sprawled in the Blue Canoe with me.

Somehow we arrive safely at the third-floor shower room. The door is opened, and I am wheeled under the shower spout. My security sheet is removed. Totally paralyzed, I lay exposed to my male and female nurses. As previously mentioned, when you check into the hospital, leave your modesty and any thought of privacy at the registration desk. Eventually a wash cloth is used to cover my privates.

Frederick checks the temperature of the water. The shower nozzle is run up and down my body, soaking me thoroughly. Just when I am about to relax, I remember the tracheotomy hole in my throat. My tracheotomy opening has not yet closed. Responding to my plea for protection, Frederick spreads a washcloth over the hole.

It is not much defense, but he promises not to let me drown. Being powerless, I take a firm seat on predestination and take pleasure from my shower.

After not bathing for half a year, I am eager to be showered. Greater than the embarrassment is the sensation of being clean. Still I am compromised. Frederick asks, "Is the water too hot? You are turning red."

"No, the water is not too hot. I am self-conscious about being naked."

Though not accustomed to having a male and female bath me, the bath is wonderful! Cleanliness is refreshing. The water running over my body is warm and soothing. I feel good, but remain anxious to be covered. Lying paralyzed, being bathed by a male and female nurse isn't my idea of a relaxing bath. Though wounded, my modesty is not dead. Still, the bath is deeply appreciated.

The Cdiff. continues to disrupt my therapy. I am cold and shivering. The diarrhea becomes worse. Medication is suspended awaiting new tests. My temperature remains abnormally high. With diarrhea I am unable to go to the pool. I am taken to the gym—not a good move. An unscheduled bowel movement prompts Rob to return me to my room.

My temperature stays at 101, with a pulse of 130. It is the weekend, the speech therapist is off-duty, so I do not eat. Halloween brings a party for staff and patients. Fearing I will have an unexpected bowel movement, I decline to go to the party. This disappoints my therapists. They in turn report to my wife I would not attend the party. With diarrhea and high temperature, I surmised I should not party. Bess becomes upset and proceeds to give me an unappreciated and undeserved lecture.

Breathing is again shallow and irregular. Bess and Diane try to encourage me to participate in all activities. I am sick and nonresponsive. Why try to explain to therapists I have fever, diarrhea, and thus feel dreadful? Again I come to realize no one really understands what another is experiencing. And once again, I resolve never to say to anyone, "I know just how you feel." Truth is, I can't comprehend how another person feels.

The next day, November 1, therapy is not possible. Dave, my respiratory therapist, is forced to put me back on the CPAP for a nap. Because of the infection and my high temperature, my air reserve and vital capacity are down. Dave does not understand why I am regressing. Again I try to go to therapy, but the diarrhea is so bad, I am returned to my room.

Things are so dark! How and when will I overcome the reoccurring problems? The temptation is to surrender, give up, quit. This I will not do. Encouragement comes from an unusual source, a poster.

166

The head nurse places on my bulletin board a placard of a football player sitting on a bench. Mud is smeared across his face and covers his uniform. His head is down and his elbows are on his knees. Tears are streaming down his cheeks. He is dispirited, discouraged, disheartened. He is defeated!

The big words underneath read, "I quit."

In the bottom corner of the poster is a picture of a rugged hill. On the hill is a cross. Underneath the cross are the words "I didn't."

I am connected to a winner, Jesus Christ! This removes the option of giving up. The assurance of the Bible is: "I can do all things through Christ who strengthens me." Daily I am putting this promise to the test of realism. Can I make it apply to a quadriplegic?

I agree with Joni Eareckson Tada, author and disability advocate, who said: "I had rather be in a wheelchair with God than on my feet without Him."

In the rehab hospital I learn when it is dark enough you see the stars. Once again I am resting on my firm faith in the goodness of God.

I often say to myself: *Things are not as bad as they seem. Things could be worse. Things will get better.* I falter when I say to myself, *Things could be worse.*

At the moment, I am not sure how, and then I remember, *I can't fall off the floor.*

# Slow, Steady Progress

*A*lthough my nerve sheath is slowly restoring itself, I am not getting a return of strength in my extremities. Weakness and lack of muscle is extreme. The respiratory therapist does not understand why I am apparently regressing.

*Does he not realize I am sick?* I wonder to myself.

He is focused only on my breathing, unaware I am incessantly battling diarrhea, a kidney infection, anxiety attacks, and fatigue. They have affected my psyche, resulting in minor depression. Every time Bess visits me, I cry.

My health is a problem. Being a major encumbrance to my wife and family poses my primary concern. Missing the babyhood years of my grandchildren is hurting. My desire is to spend time with them, play with them, and enjoy their early years. This isn't happening. Mulling this over in my mind, I become more depressed. From the day Bess and I married, family has been primary in our lives. Most troubling is not my GBS, physical weakness, or painful therapy. It is my inability to be with or help my family.

The family becomes so concerned about me they schedule a meeting on November 2 with Dr. Smith, the primary caregivers, and all my therapists. The discussion centers on their evaluation, prognosis, and future plans. It is becoming more obvious my healing is minimal.

Dr. Smith reviews my record and outlines future treatment plans. She concludes by saying, "He will recover."

Not fully satisfied, Wallace, one of my lawyer sons, asks, "To what degree will he recover? What are your long-term expectations?"

Dr. Smith replies, "The indications are Ralph should be able to transfer from a bed to a wheelchair. Much later he should walk, with a walker for support. All of these goals are *a long way off.* He will need an attendant *at all times* when he goes home. Additionally, he will need *many devices to assist him.*"

The family appreciates this honest and realistic medical evaluation. It is sobering, and helps them to more fully understand the challenges I am facing. It will be a long, hard, difficult journey back to restoration. They are encouraged, as Dr. Smith indicates I might possibly be able to go home for Thanksgiving dinner, although Christmas is more probable.

Bess relates to me the discussion and appraisal of my condition. My future does not appear very promising. The meeting probably discourages my family more than it encourages them. Nevertheless, it is good for us to understand the broad outline of the road I must travel. Our family is strong and deals well with truth.

I am elated with the possibility of a home visit on Thanksgiving. The medical evaluation that is gloomy to my family is good news to me. *Possibly I can go home for Thanksgiving dinner! Dr. Smith believes I will eventually walk on a walker!* I reason, *If I can walk on a walker, I can walk without one.*

From this evaluation meeting onward, I make steady progress. My occupational therapist attaches a strap to my right hand, to which a spoon is fixed. I attempt to feed myself. This is wasted effort. I can't lift the spoon off the table. Katie rigs a pulley-and-balance system that is attached to my forearm. Slightly lifting my hand, a counterweight raises my arm to the height of my mouth. For the first time in months, I awkwardly spoon a small portion of food into my mouth.

Bess enters the dining room just as I am making this initial attempt. It is apparent my wife is distressed that the spoon must be strapped to my hand. The balancing lift accentuates my feebleness. Tears flood her beautiful eyes. She excuses herself.

I am proud and happy to reach the point where I can attempt to feed myself. Bess loves me so much she is overwhelmed with my feeble transfer of food from dinner plate to mouth. She imagines this could be permanent.

I know it is temporary. Her beautiful heart is breaking for me. Her distress over my feebleness makes me love her all the more. My heart is rejoicing in being one step closer to independence.

My physical therapist stands me in a frame, where miraculously, I stand twenty minutes. I sit on the mat and slowly turn a bicycle peddle. On November 9, diapers become history. For the first time, on November 16, I sit on the bathroom commode. Good-bye, portable potty! I twitch all my fingers except the little finger on my left hand. My lung vital capacity reaches the 1,000 goal. The Passy Muir valve is removed from my throat. A red plug is put in the throat hole. All of a sudden, I am making great progress!

I gain strength enough to go home for Thanksgiving. Transportation is the major obstacle in my home visit. Leonard Smith makes the arrangements. He asks Bud Shivers if he can borrow his handicap van to transport me home. On Thanksgiving Robin, Bud's beautiful wife, personally drives to the hospital to transport me. This is my first home visit in eight months.

Arriving home, I see Bess has tied yellow ribbons on all the native oak trees in our front yard. As I disembark from the handicap van, I am greeted by several of our neighbors. Tears run down my cheeks. It is an emotional homecoming.

Diane and her family join us to enjoy the lunch Bess has prepared. I am in a wheelchair being fed by Bess. Still, this is the best Thanksgiving dinner in my memory, because I am home. Robin and Leonard return at 3:30 in the afternoon to take me back to the hospital. When the day ends I am happy and tired. What a wonderful Thanksgiving!

It could not have happened without Robin Shivers. I consider her to be an angel. And Leonard Smith is one of the best Christians I have ever known. For years Leonard was the personal pilot for the late Texas Governor Alan Shivers and his family. Thus he is a friend of Bud, Governor Shivers' son, and his beautiful wife Robin.

For 235 days I have been in the hospital. Dr. Smith brightens my life by telling Bess and me I am two-thirds of the way through my recovery process. After she leaves my room we spontaneously say, "Sure hope she is right!"

The hole in my throat remains completely open. When will it close? The hope is it will slowly close and heal. For the past ten days I have reverted to wearing diapers, due to the miserable Cdiff. infection. Once again, I am free of them. My pneumatologist, Doctor Mazza, is always encouraging. He says, "You are getting well and will be almost back to where you were before GBS!"

After a month's delay I receive my first pool therapy on November 28. Immediately after lunch, Frederick transfers me to my hospital bed. He removes my gym clothes and slips me into my swimsuit. Because I have lost so much weight, my swim trunks are too large. I join Frederick in laughing as I tell him, "I have never had this problem before." The waist drawstrings are tightened and I am ready for pool therapy.

Promptly at 1:00 p.m. an attendant enters my room prepared to push my wheelchair to the pool area. This area is specifically designed for handicapped patients. Water temperature is 85 to 90 degrees. As I enter the exceptionally large pool area, I am impressed by the warmth of the room. It feels like 90 degrees in there. Though I am certain it is not that warm, it is considerably higher than the 72-degree hospital temperature.

The pool is filled with people. Fifteen ladies are in a class. They are led in an exercise routine directed by a therapist. It is obvious they are enjoying themselves. Five or six hospital patients are being helped by therapists.

One end of the pool is slightly more than three-feet deep. The north end of the pool appears to be six-or-seven feet deep. The slope is gradual from end to end. There are ropes across the middle of the pool forming three lanes. On the west side of the room, near the entrance, is a treadmill submerged in the water. As I enter, seeing the treadmill, I say to myself, *Someday you will be walking on that.*

Jeff, who is to be my pool therapist, introduces himself. Six-and-a-half-feet tall, he has the body of a disciplined athlete. His blue eyes and short-blond hair make him a strikingly handsome individual. He is cordial, friendly, and possesses a winsome personality.

Introducing himself, Jeff proceeds to drape a yellow life preserver around my neck. It is secured to my chest. Wearing this erases any fear or trepidation of drowning. Additionally, a large belt is wrapped and cinched around my waist. I'm now ready for pool therapy.

Jeff gently lifts me from my chair and places me in a pool wheelchair. Made of plastic, it has unusually large wheels. With a therapist in front and behind, the wheelchair is pushed down a ramp into the pool. Having been a swimmer all my life, I find this exhilarating. It is also intimidating. I am a quadriplegic. Left to myself in the pool, I would surely drown.

I can't walk in the water—yet. The best I can do is kick ten times. After resting a minute, I kick ten more times. Additionally, I can bring my legs together in the water. A short three weeks later, with help, I stand in the pool. Water rehabilitation is the best therapy possible.

On the first day in December, I realize I will go home in a wheelchair. My goal has been to *walk* out of the hospital the day I am dismissed. I am slow to accept the reality of my continued weakness.

The Christmas season proves to be uplifting and also depressing. Christmas decorations brighten the hospital. Staff members are in a holiday mood. Their conversations indicate nearly all are going to visit family, or their relatives will visit them. Rob, Katie, and Becky take me as their guest to the hospital Christmas party. It appears I am the only patient at the party. This is making me feel very favored.

All of this Christmas festivity should lift my spirit. Instead Bess and I cry every night when we are together. We are extremely sentimental regarding Christmas. Obviously this holiday season is different. As we make plans for Christmas Eve and Day, we shed more tears.

On the evening of December 7 the Peacemakers, teenagers from our church Chapel Choir, visit. Coming into my room they serenade me with a mini-concert. What a joy to see them! As they sing, tears roll down their young faces. Having not seen me for eight months, they are shocked observing my emaciated body. None of them have seen me in a wheelchair.

December 13 proves to be another important day in my progress. Dr. Ames Smith removes the peg feeding tube from my stomach. The procedure is done in my room, and takes an hour and fifteen minutes. This same evening Bess helps me write my letter of resignation to Hyde Park Baptist Church. This letter of resignation closes over thirty-five years of ministry in a great and wonderful church.

On December 20, I stand in the pool for the first time. My therapist Jeff supports me, but **I am standing!** This weak effort opens the pathway to relearning to walk. My reasoning is: *If I am able to stand in the water, soon I can stand on land! I will one day walk.*

Two days later Dr. Ames Smith removes the catheter from my left shoulder. It has been attached to me for so many months, I scarcely realize it is there. Abnormal medical aides have become routine.

Hyde Park Baptist Church's longstanding tradition is to have a silent, candlelight, Lord's Supper Worship Service. Not a word is spoken during the entire service. It is observed on the Sunday evening closest to Christmas. Following this service hundreds of our members come to the hospital and carol. Bess and I are deeply moved by their presence. The Christmas music they sing is beautiful and heartwarming.

The next evening our deacons meet. My resignation as pastor is read. A deacon reports to Bess it is the largest deacon's meeting in the long history of our church. Many tears are shed. The resignation is official on March 19, my sixty-fifth birthday. My last paycheck from the church will be December 31.

For nine months my social life has been family visits, doctor visits, friends visiting, and hospital personnel discussing my physical needs. My social worker encourages me to broaden my social life. She tells me to get out of the hospital as often as possible.

This results in three of my therapists taking me to the Lyndon Baines Johnson Library at the University of Texas. Leonard Smith takes me to the Hyde Park Foundation Board meeting. It is a good meeting. As president of the board, I report our assets have increased over one-million dollars since our last board meeting.

A church member, while visiting me in the hospital, informs me he is making a large contribution to our church foundation. I attribute this generosity to accelerating my progress in rehab. His generosity is an uplifting inspiration to me.

My therapists, in preparing me to re-enter society, take me and three other patients to Highland Mall. The mall is adorned with beautiful decorations and filled with busy Christmas shoppers. The Christmas trees, lights, and store decorations are a cornucopia of color. This is pure fun!

Sensing this will be my only opportunity to purchase a Christmas present for my wife, I ask my therapist to roll me into a jewelry store. Carefully browsing over the ladies' jewelry section, I select a pair of large, round, gold earrings. I intend to pay with my MasterCard. Unable to hold a pen, I can't sign the charge form. My therapist volunteers to sign the MasterCard charge ticket for me.

This is the first purchase I have made in eight months. Bess will receive a Christmas present *I purchased.* My bruised ego receives healing salve with this simple transaction.

Christmas Eve and Day are happy and sad. Leonard Smith transports me home for Christmas Eve. Bess returns with me to the hospital and stays through the night. Our whole family is at our home Christmas. We enjoy a delicious lunch Bess has prepared. I am uncertain when, or how, she was able to cook lunch for the whole family.

Under our large Christmas tree are more presents than I can ever remember. Following lunch we open our gifts. Normally I distribute gifts from under the tree. My sons, Wallace and Peyton, assume my duty since I am unable to lift, hold, or even reach the presents. It is a happy and joyful time with our family.

By late afternoon I am weak from happy fatigue and return to the hospital. Alone in my room, I reflect on the day and thank God for my wonderful wife and family. Christmas is the greatest holiday of the year!

This has to be the worst and best Christmas ever. Before going to sleep I have a good long cry. I am exhilarated and exhausted.

By December 29, unassisted I am able to walk in the pool for ninety seconds. It is increasingly evident pool therapy is a vital part of my recovery process. With no fear of falling, I am able to make giant strides toward walking. The water supports my weight, a therapist holds my waist belt for support, but **I am walking!**

The New Year appears to give me new resolve and strength. Each day brings progress. I am walking further and stronger in the pool. By the middle of the month, with assistance I am walking 42 steps. January 10 brings another victory—I am able to feed myself a carton of pudding. More important is that I can do 70 percent of my transferring from bed to chair, or chair to bed. By mid-January I can walk in the pool unassisted.

My progress is slow but good. A determination needs to be made regarding my nerve return. A specialist enters my room with a fascinating electrical apparatus. I presume pods will be attached to my legs and arms. Wrong! Instead, steel needles are punched into arms and legs to determine nerve return. I have two arms and two legs. Two long slender needles are punched into each arm and leg, as tests are conducted.

This inflicts major pain. I have never had this test before. When it ends, I inform the doctor I will never subject myself to this test again. Whatever knowledge the doctor gains is not worth the severe pain I experienced.

The electric tests indicate I am getting good return to my nerves. My spirits are high! Dr. Smith believes I have no permanent damage to nerves or muscles.

Before walking I must be able to stand. For weeks my therapists have been doing everything possible to strengthen my legs. Daily strapped in the standing frame, I stand for one hour each morning. Often, if time permits, I stand in the support frame a second hour in the afternoon. Will my legs support standing without being strapped into the standing frame?

Rob pushes my wheelchair between the parallel bars. My wheelchair is elevated to its maximum height. Cautiously, I place my feet on the floor. Standing in front of me gripping the safety belt around my waist, Rob helps me stand. The wheelchair remains directly behind me. I clutch the parallel bars with arms extended for support. The therapist ceases to hold me up. I attempt to stand on land. My legs will not hold me! Except for Rob's intervention, I would be in my wheelchair, or sprawled on the floor

I am very disappointed. It is still two steps forward and one step backward.

Every Wednesday, Colleen, the psychologist, spends the hour after lunch evaluating my mental outlook. She is kind, thoughtful, and sympathetic. At first I consider these meetings unnecessary. With every passing week I have a greater appreciation of her vital role in my progress. Her questions, evaluations, and counsel encourage my recovery.

Three months have passed in rehab hospital. The realization that progress is going to be painfully slow, and sometimes not at all, is again defeating me. Some nitwit visiting me one evening remarks, "Dr. Smith, you have the rest of your life to recover." That is like throwing a drowning man an anchor. Some people would do well to never visit a patient in the hospital!

Dr. Charlotte Smith is as optimistic as ever. She continues to encourage me. She, or her partner Dr. Harris, check on me daily. Regularly they issue the therapists new treatment orders. It is increasingly evident my case is challenging the doctors and hospital staff. My therapists are concerned my leg muscles are dormant.

Every afternoon Katie attaches two electric pods to one leg, then to the other. These are attached to an E-Stem machine powered by batteries. Sending an electric current into my leg should activate leg muscles causing movement. There is no movement. Worse is the reality I cannot feel the electric current! The E-Stem is turned up high enough to leave red burns on my leg. Still I cannot feel the shock of the electrical current. The myelin sheath has not been rebuilt in my leg nerves—yet.

Doctors have assured me the myelin covering on my nerves will be restored. The rate of restoration will be approximately one inch a month. Thus in thirty-six months, the myelin covering should be restored on a thirty-six inch leg. The good news is I am short in stature, so restoration should occur sooner.

It has been nine months since I was stricken with GBS. By now there should be some significant recovery. There is little. What else can be done? Jack and Nell Brown, two of our dearest friends, provide a possible answer.

I desperately need a new approach. At this point I cry often at night when there are no visitors. I share my depressed attitude with Bess. This is unfortunate. She is suffering as much, or more, than I. During the day I am able to cope with the strenuous rehab schedule. When the rehab ends I am exhausted, and sometimes depressed.

Constantly I work on my mental attitude. Therapy is a battle that is won or lost inside the mind. Perception controls performance.

Mohammed Ali lost two fights during his career. Before both of them he said something he had not said before other fights, "If I should lose this fight ..."

We consistently act according to our beliefs. Inside my brain I must see myself walking, traveling, healed, restored! To accomplish anything I must have a goal, a hope, a dream, a vision. The Proverb writer is accurate when he writes: "Where there is no vision the people perish."

# The Hyperbaric Chamber

*J*ack and Nell Brown take Bess to dinner one evening, while I am still in NCC in Seton Hospital. Jack, a brilliant entrepreneur, has read a great deal of material regarding my illness. He is convinced that hyperbaric oxygenation possibly can enhance peripheral nerve regeneration. He explains to Bess how this perhaps can be done. At this early point in my illness the treatment can't be given, because I am on a respirator. Doctors are struggling to keep me alive.

Jack follows up on his discussion with my wife by writing this letter:

*June 6, 1995*
*Dearest Bess,*

*Regarding our discussion at dinner Friday evening, enclosed are three cards of Dr. John Lore, Medical Director of Medicine & Problem Wound Service at St. David's. Saturday afternoon I had an in-depth visit with Dr. Lore, who is quite intrigued with the possibility of enhanced peripheral nerve regeneration via Hyperbaric Oxygenation in absence of a degenerative causal agent such as MS.*

*Please do not feel any pressure whatsoever to mention Hyperbaric Oxygenation in Wednesday's meeting with all the physicians. If the situation appears proper, then proceed as you feel led.*

*As stated Friday evening, I would not have ever mentioned this possibility this early in our literature and clinical search, had it not been for the upcoming Wednesday meeting and your and everyone's increasing "desperation" to see an accelerated turnaround in the regeneration of Ralph's nerve cells.*

*The <u>very</u>, <u>very</u>, <u>very</u> last thing we would want to do at this time would be for anyone to get false hopes out of this idea. However, one would never know unless an idea is pursued. I commented to Dr. Lore, as I did to you, that it is an idea that "just won't go away." … To which he replied, "There are some ideas that should never go away."*

*Also, I would not want any of Ralph's attending physicians to get the impression that Doctor Lore is pushing himself and delving into* their *area of practice. Quite the contrary, as the advocate, I am the one to personally shoulder any blame for "meddling."*

*The idea "which won't go away" came from a discussion with Dr. Lore some time ago about Ralph's condition and whether Hyperbaric Oxygenation has ever been used to assist in the regeneration of peripheral nerves. Dr. Lore told about a rather extensive study of MS patients who received <u>temporary</u> improvements in motor functions, but no permanent improvement.*

*In reflecting upon these results, the words "temporary improvement" seemed significant.*

186

*Temporary improvement in motor function—while still in the presence of degenerative causal factor, namely MS.*

*Hence the idea/hypothesis:*

*If temporary peripheral nerve repair has been observed in the presence of the causal factor (MS) while using Hyperbaric Oxygenation, it follows that permanent peripheral nerve repair/regeneration might be achieved when the degeneration/causal factor is no longer present: e.g., in a stabilized Guillian-Barrè Syndrome patient.*

*As can be seen from the enclosed 1993 publication, animal experimentations have shown promise. Dr. Lore now has computer and telephone inquiries circulating in the "network" to determine if there are any positive clinical results with patients—where the work is in progress and yet unpublished.*

*When Ralph enters St. David's Rehab, hopefully before that time we will have obtained more definite data. Our prayer is that the Lord will reveal any such areas if it is His will for Hyperbaric Oxygenation to be one of HIS vehicles for accelerating healing of Ralph.*

*So at this point, I am reminded of someone who said, "In medicine, one should be conservative in publishing success, while at the same time being quite imaginative in making applications."*

*Jack*

One evening Bess brings Jack's letter to my hospital room and reads it to me. Neither of us have ever seen a hyperbaric chamber. We know nothing about how this treatment works, or if it will help my recovery. We do know my rehabilitation progress has been next to nothing. I am being helped by competent therapists, nurses, and staff, but *there is virtually no muscle return.* My paralysis is a tough enemy. It is not in retreat. In my quest for recovery, I am at a stalemate. The rehab automobile is locked in *park.*

Jack and Nell's encouragement and generous offer to pay for hyperbaric treatment gives me new hope. Perhaps this treatment could be the stimulus that will jump-start my nerves and muscles. With such small and slow progress, I seriously need additional help.

Before I can receive hyperbaric treatment, there is a procedure to be followed involving a considerable number of people. Substantial coordination will be necessary.

Step one involves a visit with Dr. Lore, the Medical Director of Hyperbaric Medicine at St. David's Hospital. Bess makes an appointment.

Next I ask the charge nurse's permission to leave third floor and visit Dr. Lore. Since I am still too weak to push the wheels on the wheelchair, I request a nurse to push my wheelchair from St. David's Rehabilitation Hospital to St. David's (regular) Hospital. The two hospitals are separated by a wide driveway, but connected by an underground passageway.

Before my appointment with Dr. Lore, I talk with my physiatrist, Dr. Smith, regarding the value of hyperbaric oxygenation. I secure her permission to confer with Dr. Lore regarding hyperbaric treatment. He and she will later meet and make a decision regarding hyperbaric treatment. Dr. Smith most graciously consents, with the provision it will not interfere with my daily rehab program.

Dr. Smith then concludes our discussion by saying, "Ralph, I am not sure this will help, but if I thought drinking chocolate milkshakes might help you, I would prescribe them."

Having made the necessary arrangements, on the appointed day an LVN (licensed vocational nurse) takes me to Dr. Lore's office. He is an elderly, gracious, kind, dedicated physician. He explains precisely how the hyperbaric chamber functions. With total candor, he explains he has never treated a patient with GBS, and makes no promise regarding whether the treatment will be effective in my recovery. It will be an experiment. Jack Brown's studies and enthusiasm has convinced Dr. Lore it is worth a try.

After an extensive consultation, he agrees to take me as a patient. At the end of the conference we set up a schedule for treatment. Monday through Friday, when my rehab schedule ends at 5:00 p.m., Dr. Lore will send an attendant to my room with a gurney. The attendant will transport me to the Hyperbaric Suite, where I will receive treatment. There will be thirty treatments over a six-week period. Dr. Lore emphasizes it is important not to miss any treatments. Consistency is most important!

Having made all necessary arrangements with doctors, nurses, therapists, etc., I begin hyperbaric treatment on January 18. Promptly at 5:05 p.m. a young, personable assistant to Dr. Lore enters my room pushing a gurney. I am transferred from my bed to the gurney. Five minutes later I am in the hyperbaric area

Four hyperbaric chambers are in the large room. Three are placed side by side, with the fourth across the room in a corner. Three are in use. Dr. Lore again asks if I am claustrophobic. He explains how the chamber will be filled with pure oxygen and pressurized. My ears will experience a pop similar to going up a high mountain.

I am given a large plastic container filled with water. A straw protrudes from the bottle enabling me to sip water during the treatment. Pure oxygen dehydrates the patient. Thus I am encouraged to sip on the water. Since I am incapable of holding the bottle, it is placed by my side with an extra long straw.

The intent is to saturate my body with oxygen. The treatment is one hour in length. He and I can talk with one another. During this hour I can view TV programming, or a movie. I choose 007. James Bond has always been one of my favorites. He is the only man I know who always seems to have every situation under control. Since I can control nothing, he appeals to me.

The hyperbaric chamber is similar to an elongated iron lung. It is a seven-foot steel cylinder with reinforced plexiglas on top, allowing the doctor to observe the patient. A narrow, steel, rectangular plate glides out of the cylinder. I am placed on top of the plate and slid into the cylinder. The round opening at the head of the steel cylinder is closed and hermetically sealed.

As the door of the hyperbaric chamber is shut and locked, I have a twinge of apprehension. Though I'm not prone to being claustrophobic, sealed in a steel tube is unsettling. The major danger of the treatment is fire. Special bed clothes and sheets are used. One spark in the oxygen-filled chamber could ignite me. I enter the chamber thinking, *Ralph, you could end up being burnt toast.*

Since my hyperbaric chamber treatment comes at the end of my therapy, I am exhausted. I welcome the thought of lying still for an hour. The pure oxygen, tranquil setting, and movie are relaxing to my body and weary mind. Ten minutes into my treatment I fall asleep.

At the end of the treatment Dr. Lore awakens me. He informs me pressure in the chamber is being decreased. Possibly my ears will pop. I am totally relaxed. My ears pop—close, then open. The chamber door is opened, and I am rolled out of the cylinder totally oxygenated and relaxed. Only time will disclose whether the hyperbaric treatment is effective.

Before starting hyperbaric treatment, it appears I will never use my limbs. After the second full week of treatment, I am able to slightly move my legs. Prior to this treatment my therapy results in frustration. Following the treatments my whole body seems to awaken. I am convinced the hyperbaric chamber is accelerating my progress. My medical charts indicate this treatment is a major turning point in my recovery process. Finally, my limbs are showing signs of life.

It appears my paralysis may not be permanent!

# Working toward Walking

*M*y therapists spend eight hours with me each day teaching me to walk, and use my arms and hands. My dominant concern is gaining enough strength to walk. We learn to walk as babies. Most of us walk all our lives. Walking is taken for granted. Nearly everyone walks.

I can't walk!

As Rob and I work together, he informs me I probably will not be on a walker when I am dismissed from the hospital in April. My simple response is, "Wait and see."

Truth is my hands are progressing slower than my legs. However, independent of my fingers I now move my thumbs. With my thumbs working, I am able to gain the use of my hands. Thus by January 23, I feed myself seventy percent of my lunch with a fork. The next day I feed myself all my lunch, after a therapist cuts up my chopped steak.

For the first time I feel the venodynes (compression sleeves) moving on my legs. This probably indicates the nerves in my legs are returning. Thus I walk further and stronger in the pool. On January 24, I stand between the parallel bars for thirty seconds. My legs are locked. I brace with both hands. My body is trembling, but **I am standing!**

Ever since I entered the rehab hospital, the therapists have encouraged me to push the wheels on my wheelchair. I have not had enough strength to turn the wheels. To add to my progress on this day, I push the wheels on my chair and slowly propel down the hall.

By the end of January, I have strength to do seventy-five percent of my sliding board transfers. With minimal assistance I can slide on the transfer board from bed to chair, or chair to mat, if there is no incline. More importantly, my arms are strong enough for me to put both of them around my wife. This is the first time I have been physically able to hug Bess for nine months.

I appreciate my neurologist, Dr. Michael Douglas, continuing to follow my progress and treat me. On January 29, making a routine visit, he reviews my chart and examines me. He expresses amazement at my progress. With a broad smile on his normally somber face, he says, "You will walk."

Dr. Smith adds, "Ralph, you are ahead of our projections. The therapists are doing a good job." I refrain from speaking but think, *I should be ahead of your projections. The therapists are killing me. I no longer refer to them as therapists. I call them terrorists!*

One contributing factor in my progress is the love and support I am receiving. Bess brings me a bowl of my favorite vegetable-beef soup. Two friends rent a van and take Bess and me to dinner at Trattoria Grande, my favorite restaurant. Returning to my hospital room we discover members of Young Adult 5 Sunday School Department have decorated my room with balloons and streamers. Dennis and Gloria Noble, Bess' brother and wife, drive 225 miles one-way to spend the day with Bess, and visit me. Each evening I have a number of visitors, who encourage me. To top off a great month, a friend tells Bess he has rented a handicap van for our use the next three weeks.

On the last day of the month Bess weeps, telling me she did one of the most difficult things ever. She worked from 10:00 a.m. until 5:00 p.m. packing up books in my study at church. Worse yet, she was only able to box half my books. The church has not offered me an office; consequently, we must rent storage space for my books.

Bess' tears stop when I tell her, "Honey, tomorrow they are going to teach me to brush my teeth!" This is one minuscule step in returning to normal. To me, however, it is a giant leap.

February comes with a winter breath. From my hospital room I view an icy street with virtually no traffic. Cars entering the hospital drive are slipping and sliding. Less than half of our third-floor staff are able to drive to the hospital. Bess phones leaving word she is unable to get out of our garage. The inclined drive is a sheet of snow, sleet, and ice, preventing her from leaving home.

As everyone in show business knows, "the show must go on." Thus the therapists who braved the icy streets maintain my regular regimen of therapy. With insufficient help, I complete only half my normal schedule. Because ice is covering the road the next day, followed by snow the next, my therapy is limited. I have, however, gained strength enough to stand between the parallel bars for thirty seconds.

Two goals are firmly fixed in my mind. First, I plan to be on a walker by the end of the month. Second, I promise Bess we will go to Colorado in July. Being a realist, Bess believes neither is probable. She smiles saying, "I hope so."

Dr. Smith informs me I need a $23,000 electric wheelchair. My weakness requires a chair that elevates, totally reclines, and lifts my legs. Though assigned a hospital wheelchair, I cannot use it. I have neither the strength nor the coordination to turn the wheels on a regular wheelchair. Jimmy Jackson, recently retired from the State of Texas Mental Health and Mental Retardation Commission, assures me he will try to help.

At noon the next day he reports the State of Texas will loan me an electric wheelchair. Before noon the following day, the chair is delivered.

Since I know nothing about electric wheelchairs, the employee delivering the chair explains its operation. By simply plugging into the wall socket, it can be recharged each evening. A small joystick mounted on the right arm steers the chair. Using this, the chair goes forward or backward at variable speeds. It reclines and elevates. Additionally, the leg rests can be elevated allowing me to fully recline. The turning radius is quite sharp. It is beyond anything I could imagine. I proudly tell people, "It will do anything but cook my meals."

I am intimidated by the chair. Raising my right hand to the armrest is difficult. Once it is there, I need my fingers to operate the joystick. My fingers are frail, not stable. How can I steer this heavy chair? First, I make sure the chair is turned off. Then I place the palm of my hand on the guide stick. After turning on the switch, slowly I move the stick forward at the slowest speed.

It takes me five days to feel comfortable steering the chair. During this time I accidentally back into my nurse, turn into the wall, and smash a door. The electric wheelchair provides me mobility and independence. More important is the psychological uplift I am experiencing.

The following week my OT and PT helpers inform me I need to drive the wheelchair around the St. David's Hospital block. "Gladly," is my response. They lead me to the elevator door on third floor.

"Push the elevator call button."

I try. I do not have enough finger strength to depress the elevator button. My therapist pushes the button. When we reach ground floor, the elevator door opens and I motor toward the hospital entrance doors. They open automatically. I am outside. Finding the disability ramp in the curb, I am off and rolling on the sidewalk around the buildings. My two therapists are following.

On the backside of the hospital at the garage exit, the sidewalk ends. I am forced to drive in the street. Several cars whiz by. It appears they are speeding. They aren't. I am anxious to get back on the sidewalk. With considerable nervousness, I circle the large complex, and return to the third floor. This proves to be a major breakthrough in my rehabilitation. Now I have confidence to take the chair onto the sidewalk and street. When I can transfer from my bed to the wheelchair, I will have considerable freedom.

I am as excited as a teenager with his first car. Finally, I have wheels! The electric wheelchair brings a freedom I have not experienced for ten months. Leonard Smith takes Bess and me to Luby's Cafeteria, then to a movie. Bess uses the van our friend leased, taking me for a long drive. She is driving and I am in my electric wheelchair behind her. We end the day enjoying a steak dinner at Grady's Restaurant.

One of our dear friends, W.E. (Chris) Christianson was in NCC at Seton Hospital during my stay. God called him home to Heaven. Robert, his son, visits me at the hospital to inquire if I am able to conduct Chris' funeral. After conferring with Dr. Smith and my therapists, I agree to conduct Chris' funeral. Two days later I deliver the eulogy in Hyde Park Baptist Church seated in my electric wheelchair.

Returning to the hospital, I am emotionally exhausted. I have just conducted the funeral for a great man, and a personal friend. Seeing the sorrow in his family breaks my heart. Every time I conduct a funeral, I leave a part of myself at the cemetery.

In the afternoon following the funeral, I continue my physical therapy. For two-and-a-half minutes I stand holding the parallel bars. This is five times as long as I have previously stood. I end the day happy I could bring comfort to a family, and also reach a new plateau in my standing ability.

February ends with dramatic progress. I walk across the pool in shallow water without stumbling. The pool therapist, Jeff, reports I actually am picking up my feet. Dr. Smith gives permission for me to go to Colorado in July. For the first time I am able to grasp and hold a small cup of orange juice. Finally I am able to stand between the parallel bars for five minutes.

The last day of February brings intense, painful therapy. Exhausted I am wheeled on the gurney to the hyperbaric chamber. With little success, I try to feed myself supper. I request a "no visitors" sign be placed on my hospital room door.

When Bess visits later in the evening we have a long talk regarding my condition and progress. I confess to her I am not as far along as I had hoped. My goal was to be on a walker by month's end. I am not there. I again realize it is going to be a very long time before I recover.

We hug and have a good, long cry.

Entering a new month in the rehab hospital, I remember the Bible passage: "Weeping endures for a night, but joy comes in the morning..." We had a good cry last night, but *things will get better!* They do on the first day of March. A cab that accommodates my electric wheelchair is called and delivers me to my home. A delicious T-bone steak dinner awaits me. Bess and I enjoy a quiet meal together. Though I am uncomfortable with it, Bess patiently feeds me dinner.

As we finish dinner the doorbell rings. Two couples, who are great friends, come to visit. Soon there are over twenty people in our family room! All have first gone to the hospital to visit, only to be told I am home for the evening.

After several minutes of fellowship, it is evident this is more than a friendly visit. One of the greatest friends I have, Wayne McDonald, speaks for the group. "We are your friends, we love you both. Here is a copy of a certified check for $175,000. Today the check was given to the bank paying off the mortgage on your home."

This is a complete surprise. Bess and I are overwhelmed! Speechless! Tears run down our cheeks. As best I can, I thank the group. Bess offers her thanks and appreciation, too. Now everyone in the room is wiping away tears. I know our humble thanks are inadequate, but we can't do much more. Never will we be able to adequately thank these unbelievable friends for their generosity.

Wow! What a way to start the month of March! Only a few years ago we built our home. I watched the subdivision being developed, then talked with the developer about securing a lot overlooking Lake Austin and the Hill Country.

The lots were twice what I could afford. Then our economy took a severe downturn. Because of the bad economy the developer was unable to sell lots in Lakeview II Subdivision. Consequently, the price of the lots was reduced fifty percent. Owning a home with little or no chance of selling it in the down economy, I made a down payment on my dream homesite. This required all the financial courage I could muster.

With advice and continual help from Wayne McDonald, Bess and I planned and built our new home. This would have never occurred without Don Tew designing the plans for the home at no charge, and Russell Parker building the house at his cost. One week after we moved into our new home, an attorney purchased our old house for cash, with no Realtor involved. Providence worked in our favor.

Bess and I have now been discussing our alternatives. We have lived in our new home a few years. On my retirement income, there is little, or no chance of keeping our house. It will be necessary to sell our dream home. The monthly payments are far more than my retirement income can support ... then ... our friends generously pay off our mortgage!

British poet, William Cowper, was accurate when he penned: "God moves in a mysterious way, his wonders to perform."

\* \* \* \* \*

In preparing to be released from the hospital, it is essential I courageously move back into society. My counselor is well aware of my secret fear of integrating socially. For a time, or perhaps permanently, I am a cripple. The left side of my face is partially paralyzed. When I drink, or use a straw, the liquid dribbles down my chin. I can't feed, dress, or bathe myself, or care for my toilet needs. There remain myriads of smaller physical problems.

Rob and Katie borrow the hospital van to accompany me to my home. The purpose of the home visit is to ascertain necessary changes in our house to make it handicap friendly. Even at this early date, they are preparing us for the day I will be discharged from the hospital.

Bess and I are stunned by their suggestions. Their analysis reveals we need a ramp leading to the front door. Smaller ramps should be installed in the garage and deck door. My shower stall needs to be completely remodeled, making it wheelchair friendly. This includes removing the glass door, removing the shower curb, and installing a shower chair.

Beyond this, an electric lift is needed. It will attach to a rail in the ceiling from our bed to the shower (or bathtub) and commode. A rather long list of other less expensive alterations are also connoted. Tears are flowing down Bess' cheeks. In shock, she quietly whispers, "Lord, help us."

As Rob and Katie sit at our breakfast table, they finish writing their report, and present Bess a copy. When the report is completed, I thank Rob and Katie for all they are doing to help us. Then calmly I say, "I do not believe we will need to do this, except build the ramps, remove the shower door, and purchase a shower chair."

It is obvious they are more pessimistic than I, regarding my recovery. I am convinced the key to my recovery is between my ears and in my heart. If I do not believe I will recover, I won't. Beyond faith, I need an iron will committed to whatever therapy is necessary.

This assuredly will be a long, hard, exhausting process, with no promise of success. Only time will reveal whether the therapists' proposals are essential. Even now I believe I will be able to get from my bed to the shower and toilet, etc. I could be wrong in my optimism.

As we return to the hospital, Rob and Katie are non-communicative. It is evident they believe we should hope for the best and prepare for the worst. Their observations are based on observing my age, weakness, lack of nerve return, and slow progress.

They are trained professionals doing exactly what they must. On the other hand, I am seemingly making only slow minuscule progress Yet, in my mind there is a strong belief I will recover. Just how much I'll recover remains the question.

Additionally, I must solve the transportation challenge. I have an electric wheelchair on loan. It is excessively heavy. We have been using a ramp-accessible cab or renting a handicap van. Often the van is unavailable and taxi service is undependable and expensive. There appears to be only one handicap-friendly taxi in Austin. Transportation is a problem.

The best thing about a future problem is: the future comes one day at a time. It seems useless to worry. Worrying is like sitting in a rocking chair. It gives you something to do, but it does not get you anywhere.

Bess locates a modified Dodge minivan in San Antonio. The cost is $38,184, very expensive to us. Arrangements are made to lease/purchase the van two years. The cost is $5,000 down, and $560 each month. At the end of this time we can either purchase the van, or return it. It is expensive, but necessary. It solves our transportation problem. Without it, we have no dependable means to transport the electric wheelchair.

Wayne drives Bess to San Antonio on March 14, to get the minivan. The rear passenger seats have been removed and the floor leveled. The van is equipped with an automatic back, right-sliding door. There is a ramp that electronically lowers to the ground, forming an inclined bridge from street level into the van. Once my wheelchair is inside the van, it can be secured with straps anchored to the floor. Bess can, with the click of a button, open and close the back, sliding door and lower or raise the ramp. Additionally, the door and ramp opener will start the van, allowing the vehicle to be heated, or cooled, before the passengers enter.

With the van Bess and I feel so much freedom. It is a dream-come-true. On several previous occasions we would have exited the hospital for a few hours, but no transportation was available. When I am dismissed from the hospital, and begin outpatient therapy, the van will be essential to get me to-and-from the hospital.

It was not my plan to be in the hospital on March 19, my 65th birthday. Nevertheless, here I am. I resolve to make it a memorable day. Therapists take me through my regular schedule. Nothing unusual happens until my physical therapy at 11:00 a.m.

Rob and Katie work with me in the third-floor gym. With great effort I transfer to the elevated mat. Rob proceeds to stretch my legs. As I lay flat on my back, he lifts my right leg. Katie secures my left leg with her hands. Eventually my right leg is resting on Rob's shoulder, angled forty-five degrees. I wince, shudder, and then scream in pain. The sensation is that my ligaments and muscles are tearing. Pain in my leg is searing hot.

My eyes fill with tears.

Eventually I am stretched to my limit. Rob, lowering my right leg, apologizes. He again explains, "It is necessary."

"Rob, it is OK. I am a sissy. I'll scream with pain. You keep stretching me." Then I remind Rob and Katie they are physical terrorists, not physical therapists.

They laugh with me and at me. Rob proceeds to stretch my left leg. The pain is excruciating. I scream with the searing-hot pain in my aching leg. This agonizing process is the reason many never complete remedial treatment.

*This is Pain City, USA. Happy Birthday, Ralph!*

Following the torture-chamber stretching, I transfer back to my electric wheelchair. I guide the chair to the parallel bars, parking slightly inside them. Rob attaches a wide belt around my waist. After elevating my chair, Rob holds my belt tightly, and I stand between the bars.

With arms extended and locked, I clutch the bars. Rob asks, "Can you move your right foot forward?" Slowly, I shuffle my right foot several inches forward.

Katie, with a tremor in her voice, whispers, "Try to move your left foot forward." Languidly I do.

Rob then says, "Can you do it again?" Tentatively, *I take three steps.* There is absolute silence. They encourage me to back up three steps to my chair. Eventually this is accomplished.

Fatigued, I settle back into my wheelchair. Tears are streaming down my cheeks. I whisper, "I just walked!"

Katie and Rob look at each other, and simultaneously utter, "You *are* going to walk!"

"*One* of us always knew I would walk," I retort.

"Yes, but only one …" Rob responds.

The excited discussion following led both therapists to reveal that neither believed I *would* ever walk. This, however, never prevented them, tirelessly and patiently, working to help me walk.

The Chinese proverb of Lao-tse is true: "The longest journey begins with the first step."

*Today is my 65th birthday, and I just took three steps.*

HAPPY BIRTHDAY, RALPH!!!

I take six steps on March 20, followed by ten steps the following day. Beyond that I walk ten minutes on the treadmill in the pool. These are mega-leaps in my progress. The door is open to anticipate using a walker.

From day one of my devastating GBS illness, I knew to avoid the "Blame Game." Anyone doing this is a self-pronounced victim. "Blame" is spelled b-lame. This is precisely what I am struggling not to be. I have no excuse for my illness, feebleness, or weakness. Ben Franklin said, "People who are good at making excuses are seldom good at anything else."

My responsibility continues to be to work as diligently as possible to get back to normal.

# *Walking into My Future*

*A* life-changing event is about to occur. It is Retirement Sunday. March 24 is the day I officially cease being Pastor of Hyde Park Baptist Church. For nearly thirty-six years I have had the responsibility of leading this wonderful congregation. It has been a privilege to marry young couples, visit the infirmed in hospitals, lead people to accept Jesus as Savior, baptize converts, counsel the discouraged, administer the church, conduct funerals, and preach the Bible.

Being Pastor of Hyde Park has always been exciting to me. The church has grown from a congregation of a few-hundred members to a congregation of nearly 11,000. During these years the church built eleven buildings, including a 2600-seat sanctuary. The church started a counseling center, established the Hyde Park Baptist Church Foundation, founded the Child Development Center, built an elementary and high school with 825 students, founded and built seventeen mission churches in Austin and one in Brazil.

When I would get up each morning, I could not wait to get to work. Nothing is comparable to being Pastor of

Hyde Park Baptist Church. I feel sorry for anyone who has not had the privilege of being a pastor. To me, being a pastor is fun, fulfillment, excitement, and hard work resulting in a sense of accomplishment.

My friend, Dick Rathgerber, recently taught me the formula: *S + S = C. Success plus significance equals contentment.* I have been blessed in having some success. Success is meaningless without significance. When success is linked with significance, the result is contentment. By the goodness of God, I have lived a contented, peaceful, joyful life. My hope is that my Lord is saying, "Well done, good and faithful servant."

This takes the sadness from Retirement Sunday. I have done my best to be a faithful servant-pastor at Hyde Park Baptist Church. Now I am entering another chapter in my *Book of Life.* Hopefully, the best is yet to be. I have often prayed, "Lord, let me live in such a way that when I die, even the funeral director will be sad."

As I come to deliver my final sermon at Hyde Park, the church is filled with chairs down the aisles, around the walls, and in the balcony. An overflow crowd is watching on closed-circuit TV in our Fellowship and Friendship Halls. I am especially pleased that many of the St. David's Hospital rehabilitation staff are present. Without them I would not be speaking today.

A ramp has been built leading up to the first level of the rostrum in the sanctuary. This allows my electric wheelchair to move up to viewing level for the congregation. My granddaughter Lisa sings one of my favorite songs. The choir, led by Joe Carrell, our minister of music, is superb. Madison, my seven-year-old grandson, and Chandler Jones, age eight, read from Romans chapter eight, the Bible text for today's message, "More Than Conquerors."

My sweet wife Bess speaks to the congregation. Her eloquence, sincerity, and message brings tears to my eyes. She concludes by quoting from *Camelot*. In her memory, being at Hyde Park is comparable to being at Camelot.

Following my sermon, scores of members and guests speak to us expressing love and appreciation. We are deeply touched and emotionally exhausted. We go to our home and enjoy a delicious lunch with our whole family.

I am thankful for Retirement Sunday for several reasons. First, I have lived long enough to retire. Some do not have this opportunity. Additionally, the church is large, strong, and healthy. Bess and I have anticipated this phase of life. Fortunately, my identity is not just in my work as pastor. I have many other interests and happily anticipate retirement.

\* \* \* \* \*

The week following Retirement Sunday is marked with progress in therapy and fun in my social life. One day my therapists permit me to attend the citizens' board meeting at the Austin Country Club. On Saturday, Bess and I watch our grandson Jeff play baseball. Following the game we take in a movie. This same week we go to a University of Texas baseball game. Sunday we attend church as regular members, not pastor and first lady.

To every action there is a reaction. For the past week my schedule has been strenuous therapy followed by a busy, happy social life. I'm exhausted.

Katie enters my room Monday to stretch my arms and fingers. I am still in bed and do not want to get up. The Second Law of Thermodynamics is true. Like the universe, I am running down.

Katie, who now is a personal friend as well as therapist says, "You are too tired to do therapy, aren't you?"

"Yes," is my meek response. I am ashamed of myself, but too exhausted to tackle my daily therapy routine. She exits, seemingly frustrated.

After a time Katie returns. My thought is, *She is going to say get yourself up and out of that bed!* Instead she utters, "I have talked with your doctor. There will be no therapy today. We want you to rest." Whether she is pouting or relieved, I am unable to discern. Whatever her disposition, she just made me extremely happy. This is day 356 in the hospital. I *am* exhausted, wiped out, frayed, tired, and beyond the point of going. A rest day is essential to my psyche. Somerset Maugham well expressed what I am experiencing. "Only mediocre people are always at their best."

"Upward and onward" is my theme the following day. The day in bed proved to be exactly what my body needed. After lunch, unassisted I walk 165 steps in the shallow end of the pool. This new record is a harbinger indicating eventually I will walk without the buoyancy of water. Pool exercise continues to be the most productive therapy. In the final therapy session of the day, I stand for fifteen of the longest minutes of my life, between the parallel bars. This is another new record in my struggle towards normality.

Progress during April is most encouraging. On April 5, using a walker I walk twenty feet. By April 19, I am able to walk thirty-nine feet.

Perhaps "shuffling" better describes my walking. With both hands resting on the walker (I can't actually grasp it yet), keeping my legs locked and stiff, I lift one foot then the other. If I attempt to bend my knees in walking, I sink. Thank God, Rob is there to catch me, or I would be on the floor. My knees are not yet strong enough to support me, thus I keep both legs locked when walking.

Nevertheless, I am walking!

I have consistently believed my foremost task is regaining the strength and ability to walk. It now appears my hands and fingers pose the greater challenge. With stiff fingers, and virtually no grip strength, I can hardly hold anything. Though Dr. Smith assures me my hands are coming back, I am essentially unable to use them. How do I grasp a glass? Just like a toddler, with two hands.

My great friend, Ed Perry, is sympathetic about my problem. During his visits I have related to him my perplexity of not being able to talk on the phone, because I can't grip a phone. On one of his visits he gives me a new speakerphone. With it, all I need to do is press a button and talk.

This is not as easy as it appears. My fingers are not strong enough to press the answer button. After a time I solve the problem. I am able to press my fist on the button. Finally, I can receive calls from my wife, family, and friends. Thank you, Mr. Alexander Graham Bell! It has been a year since I have used a telephone.

I am becoming comfortable with the electric wheelchair. With it, and the handicap van, Bess and I have great mobility. She picks me up at the hospital and we go to a movie.

214

\* \* \* \* \*

On one day, after going to the movie, when Bess returns home she becomes very sick with severe cramps. She phones our daughter for help. Diane comes and drives her to the hospital emergency room at St. David's.

The medical staff soon diagnoses that she is having a gallbladder attack. During the night her gallbladder is removed. When I awaken the next morning I am told of her emergency operation.

Now we are both in the hospital!

With the charge nurse's permission, I drive my electric wheelchair from the Rehabilitation Hospital to St. David's Hospital to visit Bess. We are a pathetic couple. She is recovering from surgery, and I am in a wheelchair convalescing from GBS.

As I visit, it is all I can do to refrain from crying. I've come to encourage my wife. Tears are discouraging. Observing she is in pain, I make my visit brief. I pray for her and exit. In the hall tears flood my eyes and roll down my cheeks. By the time I return to my room I have regained my composure.

*Things are not as bad as they seem. Things could get worse. Things will get better. We can't fall off the floor.*

After lunch, I am permitted to visit Bess again. She is woozy and apparently very uncomfortable. The visit goes better, but I remain very distressed. My wife has been helping me for a year during my illness. Now she needs help, and I can't assist her. All I can do is be by her side, as often as my schedule allows.

April 16, the next day, is our son Wallace's birthday. Bess is still in the hospital recovering. Her temperature remains elevated. She is concerned it is our son's birthday. She needs to be concerned about recovering! The best I can do is phone Wallace and wish him a happy birthday.

On April 17 Diane checks Bess out of the hospital and drives her home. Since Diane is teaching school, Bess is home alone. I worry about her recovering from surgery with no one at home to help her. I think, *Surely, someone from our church will offer to be with Bess. The church will check on her.* This does not happen...I am helpless to do anything except pray for her.

On Sunday, Jimmy Jackson drives to our home, gets the van, drives to the hospital, and takes me home for the day. Bess is still convalescing, but greatly improved—*things will get better.* Late in the afternoon Jimmy comes to our home, returns me to the hospital, drives back to my house to return the van. What a great friend! By day's end he must have thought he was a taxi driver.

Dr. Smith informs me I can be released from the hospital in a few weeks. For over a year I have been hospitalized. Here highly trained nurses, doctors, therapists, and staff have cared for me. At home Bess will be my main, and perhaps only, caregiver. This is too much to ask of my wife. Dr. Smith has indicated I will need a professional caregiver.

I have made and am making steady progress. Yet, I am incapable of performing essential functions. I am unable to totally feed myself. It is necessary for a helper to bathe me, and assist with my toilet needs. I can neither hold a urinal, nor clean myself. With great effort I can sit up on the mat or bed. If I fall to the floor, I can't get up. My hands are not flexible or strong enough to hold a glass, phone, toothbrush, or open a door.

I am still a helpless, dependent cripple.

Without a caregiver, I know Bess and I cannot make it. Bess is contending with her old nemeses, blood clots. The week following her surgery she suffered with a clot in her left leg, causing fever. She is not in the best of health. Needless to say, neither am I. Going home may prove to be more challenging than being in the hospital.

I am nervous.

On May 3, using the walker, I walk from the gym to the nurses' station. This is 149 feet! People are standing in the hall applauding and cheering, as I reach the nurses' station. Most of the staff were convinced I would never walk again. I believe they are applauding for themselves as well as for me. My walking would never have occurred without their diligent work and encouragement.

On May 13, I practice transferring on the sliding board from a quickie wheelchair to Bess' car. Amazingly I am able to do this with little difficulty. For the first time, Bess sees me walk the length of the hallway. Rob is holding the safety belt around my waist in case I stumble, or my strength fails. Katie is right behind me with my electric wheelchair.

As I continue to improve, Bess and I are able to go out-and-about enjoying friends and family. Friends drive us to Dock's in Marble Falls for a delicious catfish dinner. Additionally, I conduct a wedding in the chapel at Hyde Park Baptist Church followed with a reception dinner at El Rancho.

Wallace and his family take us to lunch on Mother's Day. Wallace, Lanette, and their three children are superb hosts. They honor Bess, give her a gift, and everything is perfect. Then our meal is served. The luncheon turns sour.

Attached to my right arm is a leather device secured by Velcro. A fork is placed in this device allowing me to feed myself. I am extremely proud I am now able, clumsily, to fork food into my mouth. It has taken me six months of rehab to get to this point of recovery. I can feed myself with approximately the skill of a clumsy three-year-old child.

218

Unfortunately, I spill some of my food during the transfer from plate-to fork-to mouth. This embarrasses Bess. She decides to feed me. I am offended by her negative reaction to my clumsy technique. As is often the case, we have two perspectives regarding my eating.

When the meal ends we thank Wallace, Lanette, and grandchildren for the delicious lunch. Bess intends to drive me home for the afternoon. Still chafing over her criticism of my attempts to feed myself, I tell her to return me to the hospital.

I am extremely proud of being able to feed myself, however clumsily. She should not have been embarrassed. I should not have become irate. We are both wrong. We are both right. Our emotions are fragile. It's okay. Bess and I have the grace to forgive and forget. Neither of us is prone to become historical—remembering past disagreements. I still think she is perfect.

The long-anticipated day finally arrives. Homecoming is May 15. Frederick dresses me. Following breakfast my belongings are assembled. Bess checks me out of the rehabilitation hospital. Two nurses accompany Bess and me, as we depart from Room 300. Tears are streaming down my cheeks as I say farewell to my nurses and attendants. They have been magnificent helpers and encouragers for the past six months. I am indebted to each of them.

As I guide my electric wheelchair toward the hospital entrance, I view a large crowd at the door. Several of our church staff and secretaries have come to the hospital with balloons, ribbons, and other paraphernalia expressing celebration. Indeed, this is one of the happiest days of my life.

While I wheel toward the minivan the host of friends sing, "This is the day the Lord has made, we will rejoice and be glad in it."

This is one of my favorite verses of scripture. Awakening each morning, this is the scripture I quote to myself. It always strengthens me.

Arriving home Bess and I are greeted by a throng of couples. This is the group that paid off the mortgage on our home. We are deeply touched. Tears well up in our eyes, coursing down our cheeks. Bess has yellow ribbons tied to all the oak trees in our front yard. What a joyful homecoming!

For the first time in thirteen months, we go to bed together. Both of us sleep like babies. God is good. Our prayer is we will have many more years of joy together. The challenge of total, or at least more, recovery lies before us.

# Finish It!

To be home is wonderful! The problem Bess faces is meeting the needs of a paralyzed husband. I have made extremely slow progress toward recovery. My challenge is to become self-sufficient. Myriads of physical challenges remain. It is evident I am doing good. Yet, currently I am good for nothing!

Without help I cannot transfer from our bed to my wheelchair, or from the wheelchair to the toilet or shower. Strength and skill are still lacking to dress myself. I lack the strength to open a door, hold a glass of water, or even press our doorbell. I remain virtually helpless. Bess is the caregiver.

When I entered the rehabilitation hospital, Dr. Smith carefully explained to our family, after coming home I will still need skilled help. Securing the names of several professional caregiver services, Bess calls one for assistance. She enlists the aid of a male caregiver. The next day he arrives at our home at 8:00 a.m.

His duties are to assist me getting out of bed, eating breakfast, getting on and off the toilet, showering, shaving, brushing teeth, etc. He then gets me dressed for the day. His morning responsibilities completed, he departs at 10:00 a.m. Returning at 4:00 p.m he prepares me for the evening. After several days we realize it will not be necessary for the caregiver to assist in the afternoon.

Our attendant works four days, but doesn't show up on day five. Nothing is one-hundred percent. Bess contacts the company and secures another aide. Though she is somewhat incompetent, we continue to employ her for a week. She also fails to appear one morning. Finding someone reliable is difficult. It is essential I have help in the morning.

This is putting a major strain on Bess. From my standpoint, I refuse to continue allowing Bess to take care of my toilet needs. I reason, this alone can ruin a good marriage.

Eventually, God sends Renee to be my caregiver. She is gentle, sweet, personable, kind, and most important of all, dependable. Renee is beautiful enough to be a movie star. After being with us three days, she is like a family member. The Bible states some "entertained angels unawares." Renee is our angel. Until I no longer require a caregiver, she helps me.

Realizing our home must be modified to meet my needs, several changes are made. Bess has the shower glass door replaced with a plastic curtain. With the larger opening, it is possible for me to transfer with assistance from my wheelchair to the shower chair. This chair can also be placed over the commode.

A long ramp that extends from our walkway to the front door has previously been installed. A shorter ramp is purchased, giving me access to our back deck overlooking the hills and Lake Austin. Our garage is separated from our house by a breezeway. Lyle Blackwood graciously builds a short ramp to accommodate the electric wheelchair entering the back of the garage. Additionally, he builds a small ramp for the step-down inside the garage. These four ramps provide me accessibility to our home, garage, front yard, and back deck.

Mountain Villa Drive is the street on which we live, indicating we live on a mountain. In Texas every hill is a mountain, every creek a roaring river, every hole in the ground an oil well ... and every man a liar. Since our home is on a steep slope, it is split-level. We have a large back deck overlooking the Hill Country and Lake Austin (Colorado River). I am unable to go downstairs to the study, a bedroom, game room, sunroom, and pool area.

Summer has just arrived. Our children and grandchildren visit often. This is a happy time as the family gathers downstairs around our pool and spa. I guide my wheelchair onto the upper back deck and watch the children splash and swim below. I yearn to be in the pool with them. I can see them, hear them, and even join in conversation with the family. This is a happy time. Often it is also a sad time for me.

After they leave, I sit in my wheelchair on the back deck. Tears well up in my eyes. I wish I could be downstairs, on the deck, and with them in the pool. I've been with them, yet I've been removed from them. This makes me more determined than ever to acquire enough strength to go up and down our stairs, get in the pool, and swim with my grandchildren.

Sitting on the deck I reflect on the thirteen months spent in the hospital. *Thank God for the progress I have made. Yet, there is still so far to go before I can walk, travel, and get in the pool with my family. Seemingly my needs are endless. I am struggling to maintain my composure. I still have little control over my life. I remain essentially helpless. Before me are many months of outpatient therapy.*

*How do I continue to cope with the seemingly endless challenges ahead? I must not dwell on my weak condition. Is there some technique I can devise to preserve me from continually mentally dwelling on my frail physical condition? How do I avoid depression?*

The answer is to have a "Pity Party."

It appears contradictory, but a principal method I employ to overcome my depressed spirit is to give myself a Pity Party. I find it effective only if I know when to end the party. In fact this is the reason to have a Pity Party. I limit my sadness to a specific time frame. Here are the components I employ to produce a successful and productive Pity Party.

**Step one:** *I am the only person present.* I "enjoy" the party alone. If I share it with another, he or she will not understand, and I will not get the full benefit of my party.

I often think of the man who asks a friend, "Have I ever told you about my operation?"

The friend responds, "No, and I really do appreciate it."

Weeks ago I realized the world isn't interested in my illness, struggles, and continued weakness.

**Step two:** *Mentally I list every problem I have, or think I might have in the future.* I recall all the pain, problems, troubles, and frustrations I am enduring. Then I meditate on them. I recognize that some of the problems will be with me the remainder of my life. I am totally absorbed in the seemingly impossible challenges before me.

The reason this is so beneficial is because I can't fall off the floor. Usually, we don't come up until we hit the bottom. I am at the bottom. Pondering my options, two poor scenarios are etched in my mind. I can remain virtually a quadriplegic. My fate will thus confine me to a wheelchair, bed, and eventually a nursing home. The second option is death. For many days during the early phase of my Guillian-Barrè Syndrome, I earnestly prayed to die. To me that would have been preferable to languishing in the "vegetable-person" category I endured in NCC. At that time death would have been a welcome relief. Thankfully, I have moved beyond this illogical and depressed state of mind.

**Step three:** *A good long cry.* Eyes are the windows of the soul. Tears can wash these windows sparkling clean. Crying is therapeutic. Tears release tension that strangles the mind. Sorrow is a disease for which every patient must treat himself. I am not ashamed to rely on *tear pills.*

If Moses the great lawgiver, could weep, and David the great king, shed tears, then crying must not be considered weakness, but rather strength. It is the mark of our humanity. Machines do not shed tears.

The shortest verse in the Bible states: "Jesus wept." Surely, if the divine Son of God unashamedly wept, I can also. Tears are a gift from God that strengthens the inner self. They are a release valve to protect my psyche.

I know my Pity Party is off to a good start when my heart beats faster, my mind is overwhelmed with my problems, and tears are flowing down my cheeks.

**Step four:** *I reduce my problems to one written sentence.* This is one essential antidote to worry. Years ago I learned to never worry about anything until I took the time to write my problem down in one sentence. This step poses a major challenge to me. Paralyzed, I can't write. Unable to write, I stamp my problem in my mind. Here it is: *I am paralyzed, could remain a virtual quadriplegic, and may be in a wheelchair the remainder of my life.*

**Step five:** *I humbly talk to God.* I tell Him I am overwhelmed. I open my heart admitting my weakness and need for power beyond my own. I am not reluctant to state my frustration. Some might advocate talking with God as the first step. This appears ideal. In the reality of my experience, however, it works for me as step five.

It isn't wrong to ask, "Why did this happen to me?" When Jesus was nailed to the cross he prayed and asked, "My God, My God, why have you forsaken me?"

If I ask "Why?" I probably will not get an answer to this profound question. If I did get an answer, would it really help? I refuse to ask, "Why I am paralyzed?" As before-mentioned, if I knew the answer, it would not facilitate my recovery.

While going through outpatient therapy, I fall. Pain in my ankle is severe. I go to Dr. Bob Dennison, an orthopedic surgeon. An x-ray is taken and shortly thereafter, Dr. Dennison examines my ankle. He explains I have a broken (cracked) ankle. He goes on to elucidate they will make a walking cast. Wearing it, I will heal in eight-to-ten weeks. I am encouraged and satisfied. The healing occurs as he predicts.

Dr. Dennison is a wise and skilled physician. He could have explained how ankles operate. No doubt, he could have shared considerable medical terminology regarding my leg, ankle, foot, and bone structure. He could have lectured me on being more cautious. Instead, he simply put my ankle in a cast and told me I would heal.

Truth is, I would not have understood a medical explanation. All I need to know is I will get well. The same principle applies to problems I face in life. I do not need explanation. I need faith and assurance that I will get better, or at least survive. Beyond that, I need assurance that even death means I simply move from life on earth to a better life in Heaven.

**Step six:** *I end my Pity Party* by asking myself three questions.

1. What can I do to help myself?

2. What can others (family, friends, professionals) do to help me?

3. What can only God do to solve my problem?

The order is a fixed law for solving seemingly imposs-ible problems. Use all available help, then seek God's help and guidance. He is always our greatest resource!

Years ago in *Reader's Digest*, I read an interesting article. As I remember, the three pages were entitled, "Making a Graceful Exit," or something like that. The article made a profound impression on my young mind. The writer re-lated how guests would exit his home saying, "I have to go!" They say "good-bye," gather their belongings, purses, coats, etc., walk to the front door, open it, and stand in the doorway thirty more minutes talking. The host stands with them, feeling the air conditioning leave and seeing the flies and mosquitoes enter. Other guests are neglected because those departing did not leave.

Some people stay longer in an hour, than others in a week!

In contrast, the writer told of a departing guest who said, "I had a delightful time." Then he got up from his chair and promptly departed.

**My Pity Party is over**. *Ralph, get up and leave it behind!* If it is necessary, I can have another Pity Party tomor-row, but *no more moping around today!* I am learning when life throws me a knife there are two ways to catch it—by the blade or by the handle.

With this simple plan I avoid being depressed *all the time*. I have limited my depression to a few minutes, that is a "party." It is a giant step toward recovery when I turn my darkest hour of depression into a party.

There is a stress-relieving principle involved. In my ministry I did a great deal of marriage counseling. It was common to couples to say, "We quarrel often. What can we do?"

My answer was, "Have a fuss day. Just as you have a day to shop, mow the lawn, go to church, etc., have a day to argue. Set one day aside each week to quarrel. Agree not to get into conflict on any other day." Sounds silly, but it works!

This is why I have a Pity Party. I set a time to really wallow in my troubles—get depressed, mope, moan, cry, pity myself. When the party is over, I refuse to think about my problems anymore that day. This approach consistently delivers me from the dark pit of depression. Yes, I do have depressing times, but I am not a depressed person.

In fact, I have some hilarious times at my Pity Parties. I've been lower than the floor, down in the basement, buried in melancholia. But when the party is over, I leave. More important, I leave my problems also.

William James accurately wrote: "The greatest discovery of my generation is that human beings can alter their lives by altering their attitude of mind." Right in the midst of my weakness and frustration, I am having a pleasant time with my mind, for it is happy.

With great effort, I am barely moving my arms and legs. Stiff and weak, my fingers remain virtually useless. I am unable to bend my wrists or move my toes. There is no planter or pickup flexion in my feet. As I remind myself *I have little strength,* the words of Victor Hugo resonate in my mind: "People do not lack strength, they lack will."

Additional professional help is essential to my recovery. Bess drives me to St. David's Rehabilitation Hospital. We complete the necessary papers for outpatient therapy. Prior to my arrival Dr. Smith has arranged my schedule. Sessions will be Monday, Wednesday, Thursday.

| | |
|---|---|
| Physical Therapy | 11:00 a.m. |
| Lunch | Noon |
| Occupational Therapy | 1:00 p.m. |
| Pool Therapy | 2:00 p.m. |

The schedule appears simple. To us it is a challenge. I must leave our home before 10:30 a.m. three days a week. I will not return home until after 4:00 p.m. Three days each week, Bess will be making two round-trips to the hospital. This is a drive time of two hours Monday, Wednesday, and Thursday.

A wonderful friend, Jimmy Jackson, visits me. He inquires about my outpatient therapy and offers to help anyway he can. Having retired from his executive position with the state, he volunteers to drive me back and forth to therapy. What a relief to my precious wife!

In the ensuing weeks Jimmy faithfully arrives at our home at 10:15 a.m. on Monday, Wednesday, and Thursday, and drives me to the hospital. He picks me up at 3:45 to 4:00 in the afternoon to drive me home. After a week, I realize Jimmy is returning the van to my home, getting his car, then returning in the afternoon to get the van. I ask him to please keep the van while I am in therapy. If he needs to go anywhere, use the van. Reluctantly, he agrees. He is doing so much to help us.

Knowing he will soon move to Tyler, Texas, Jimmy enlists several friends to drive me to-and-from the hospital. Oscar Kellner (now deceased) assumes Jimmy's role in driving. Unselfishly, he helps me for months. Jimmy and Oscar are two of God's choice servants.

Hearing of my need to go back and forth to rehab, several other friends volunteer to be drivers. Among those who help are Lyle Blackwood, Leon Manly, Eldon Bebee, Wayne McDonald, Louie Raven, Rogers Wilson, and others.

Words can't adequately express the assistance these men are to Bess and me. Visiting with them as they drive me to therapy proves to be uplifting. My world has shrunk to the narrowness of self-preservation. Unknown to them, these men became counselors and encouragers. Additionally, they are keeping me abreast with sports, mutual friends, church, and society happenings. Driving back and forth is the highlight of my day.

Though familiar with the rehab process, I am not prepared for the intensity of outpatient therapy. It is my first day and I arrive at the hospital at 11:00 a.m. I report to the hospitality desk and await my therapist. Shortly after my arrival, Greg appears, we introduce ourselves, and he leads me to the gym. It is a large carpeted area filled with all manner of equipment for the physically challenged. In the south and north ends of the room are two areas cordoned off with sliding drapes. These areas are divided into three smaller areas used for evaluations and conferences. They afford a *small* measure of privacy.

We go to one of these smaller areas. As do all the therapists, he begins with strength measurement and evaluation. Following this very detailed procedure, goals are established. This consumes most of my hour (really it is 50 minutes) designated for physical therapy. For the final ten minutes Greg seats me on the leg exerciser. Here I pump my legs up and down. With limited resistance on the machine, I sustain the leg pumping eight minutes.

It is noon. The plan is for me to eat in the hospital cafeteria. How? Greg accompanies me to the cafeteria. He graciously introduces me to the cafeteria director. She volunteers to get someone to assist me when I come to the cafeteria. Greg informs me that going to lunch, getting my food, and feeding myself is an important part of rehabilitation.

My second day in outpatient therapy, I go unaccompanied to the cafeteria. As promised, the cafeteria director helps me get lunch. I wheel over to a table and eat lunch. *I can go to lunch alone! Wow!*

Following lunch, I guide my electric wheelchair back to the hospital reception area. In a few minutes Mark greets me. He is my occupational therapist. As always, we begin with an evaluation. Goals are established. In the remaining minutes Mark dips my hands in hot wax, wraps them in Saran Wrap and towels. Following this he bends and stretches my fingers.

Promptly at 2:00 p.m. Greg appears again informing me he will be my pool therapist. Taking me to the men's dressing area, he assists me in taking off my shoes, socks, shirt, and gym pants. Anticipating pool therapy, I am wearing bathing trunks under my pants. We spend a delightful hour in the pool kicking, stretching, walking, and deep walking. Pool therapy is the least taxing exercise and the most productive. I now am able to walk in the pool unassisted. On the pool treadmill I walk rapidly for ten minutes. I have stamina to walk much longer but others are waiting to use the treadmill.

My first day in outpatient therapy is most productive. I am exhausted and anxious to go home. Greg escorts me back to the gym, assists me in transferring to the mat, places my clothes near me, and informs me I need to get dressed.

"Greg, I can't dress myself!"

"Do the best you can. I will be back to help you with what you cannot do." Drawing the white drape around the mat, he exits.

My immediate challenge is getting out of a wet bathing suit. With considerable effort I wiggle out of the trunks. Step two is getting into my underwear. Dropping my boxer briefs on the floor, I place my feet in the leg openings. It is a tough struggle pulling up my underwear. My thumb and fingers are too weak and inflexible to grasp the elastic band and pull up. Eventually I get the boxer shorts to my hips. Since I can't stand to pull up my briefs, I roll onto the mat and wiggle into the underwear.

*So what if my briefs are crooked? I put them on!*

I try to put on socks. With no gripping strength, it is futile. Getting my arms through the sleeves, I pull my golf shirt over my head. Now comes the difficult task of pulling the shirt down. Once again I am confronted with how essential is pinching strength in my fingers. Little by little I unroll the shirt, bringing it down inch by inch to my waist.

Dropping my gym pants on the floor, I place my legs in the openings. The process used in getting into my underwear is repeated. Minus shoes and socks, I am dressed. I am also soaking wet with sweat. Yes, I know a horse *sweats* and a person *perspires*. Well, I've been working like a horse. Every step of my progress toward recovery is a sacrifice.

Rolling over and stretching out on the mat, I begin to chuckle. *What a great first day! I can go to the cafeteria, get my lunch (with assistance), feed myself, and almost dress myself. If everyday brings this much progress, it won't be long before I am independent again.*

Wrong!

Progress is at the speed of a slow snail plodding through hills of mud. It requires eight months after being dismissed from the hospital to attain these functional improvements:

Open doorknob at home with right hand

236

Manipulate utensils with right hand, except knife

Lift commode top and flush

Push elevator buttons

Use electric razor

Manipulate toothbrush

Hold newspaper and turn pages

Open sugar packets with teeth and bilateral hands

Hold toilet paper for bowel hygiene

Toilet with walker

Manipulate finger foods (e.g. popcorn and sandwiches)

Take coat off hanger while standing

Click computer mouse

Open refrigerator

Buckle seat belt

Hold in one hand a third-full soda can

I am like a child awakening daily into a new world. It is as if my body has been sleeping. I can see the dawning of a new and different life. My life is going to be as good as I make it. Good is done by degrees. All I can do is my best, that's bad enough. Wise old Samuel Johnson wrote: "The future is bought with the present." It is apparent I am going to get as well as I work to become.

My wrist movement is a major cause of concern. Both wrists remain stiff, inflexible, and hinder the use of my hands. I determine to work diligently on releasing my stiff wrists. How? Placing my right hand on the breakfast table, I wedge my left hand under my right hand. Ten times I lift my right wrist with my left hand. Switching hands I repeat the process.

This process is repeated eight or more times daily. After six months I am able to lift each wrist. Similar procedures are employed rehabilitating other parts of my anatomy. If I live long enough, and persistently work at rehab, I will recover.

Wanting desperately to walk, I ask Chad McMillan, former University of Texas football player, to help me. Chad responds, "If you will teach me theology, I will help you learn to walk." In the ensuing weeks Chad comes to our home in the afternoons, wraps a belt around my waist, which he grips in case I fall. Together we walk the back, upper deck of my house.

The deck overlooking Lake Austin is about eighty feet in length. On first attempt I walk halfway and, exhausted, return to my wheelchair. In three months, unassisted, I am able to walk the deck from end to end. In six months I can walk the length of the deck twenty times.

One major obstacle remains regarding my ability to enjoy our home. I am too weak to go up and down our stairs. This keeps me from the bottom level of our house where the game room, exercise bike, and my study are located. Additionally, I can't access the spa and pool. I absolutely must be able to get up and down our stairs! How?

Rob, my therapist during my six months in the rehabilitation hospital, volunteers to come to our home on Saturdays. He gives me additional help in learning to walk better and to get up and down our stairs

Additionally, I hire a hospital aide to come to my home on his day off and teach me to walk up and down the stairs. For the first time I am frightened. Walking up and down stairs is dangerous. One misstep and I will have a broken leg, pelvis, or head injury. Falling is something I must avoid.

Eighteen months after being dismissed from the hospital, I walk down our stairs and enter the spa. No real problem—it took only thirty-one months from the date I entered the hospital. Years ago I learned that no challenge is too great for the person who advances deliberately. *I am going to walk out of my paralysis!*

During these eighteen months I am still going to therapy three days each week. Under the guidance of Lanell, my therapist, my strength and endurance are increasing. Using a bed or chair, I stand up from the floor. With no arm push, I stand up from a nineteen-inch chair. I continue to use my walker, but am progressively using a cane. Finally I can walk into the shower and hold a bar of soap with one hand. I am able to care for all my bathroom needs.

A friend asks me what I learned from my illness. I answer, "Don't get sick!"

I keep remembering, not *what*, but *who* got me through my GBS. God, wife, family, friends, nurses, therapists, doctors, and a host of others brought me from down-and-out, to up-and-around. I can never thank each of you enough. If you meet a quadriplegic who is now walking, he did not do it alone.

Things are never as bad as they seem. They could get worse. They will get better.

Success, or failure, is never final. There is no place at which, having arrived, we can remain. I get up each morning saying to myself: *This is the day the Lord has made, I will rejoice and be glad in it.*

Life is good and always getting better.

# *Epilogue*

*T*en years have elapsed since the onset of my Guillian-Barrè Syndrome illness. When I began writing this book I could not hold a pen, and did not own a computer. A computer would not have helped. My fingers were incapable of typing. Even using the hunt-and-peck method was out of the question. I did not have the finger strength to push the keys. I longed to write a book that would be encouraging, helpful, and inspirational. My weakness made this dream seemingly impossible.

My precious friend, Jack Brown, gave me a computer as a retirement gift from the church. He then employed a computer technician to install Dragon Dictate in my new computer. Since I am computer illiterate, she taught me how to use this voice-activated program. Sitting in my electric wheelchair, talking to my computer, I began writing this book. "Scratch that" became the command used most often in voice dictation. Though mistakes were abundant, I began to write (dictate) the book.

The book should have been completed in a year. Two things hindered my writing. First, I was going to therapy three days a week, doing therapy at home, and imposing on friends to help me learn to walk on our back deck. Physically I was exhausted at the end, and sometimes middle, of the day. Second, writing this has been mentally painful. It is not pleasant recalling weeks struggling to breathe on a respirator. Recalling events in the rehabilitation hospital brought mental pain. What occurred in therapy, I wanted to forget.

It is difficult to write a book when your eyes are clouded with tears. Attempting to describe my hospital experiences, I often became overwhelmed. Then I found myself not being mentally tough enough to recall the frustration experienced during my thirteen months in Seton and St. David's Hospitals.

Understand, the frustration relates to me, not the hospitals or hospital personnel. No patient could have better treatment than I received. Without the professional care of the nurses, therapists, staff, and doctors, I would be dead. I remain amazed they could keep me alive and then rehabilitate me back to near normal. The reality is, I either should be dead, or sitting in a wheelchair, paralyzed permanently.

Having explained my delay in writing, I state without reservation, or mental hesitation, this decade of my life has been beyond belief. Life is wonderful!

This is not to infer I have no problems—I mean opportunities. Foot drop is a nuisance. Using light AFO's (ankle-foot orthoses [brace]) solves my inability to lift my toes. Titanium soles slip into my shoes, lifting my toes. This allows my walking gate to be almost normal.

My quest to become stronger, mobile, and enjoy a normal lifestyle is amazingly successful. Arriving home in an electric wheelchair, I soon progressed to a walker, then a Canadian crutch. Eighteen months after my dismissal from the rehabilitation hospital, I was able to walk from my car into outpatient therapy, using only a cane. By this time I have given away my walker.

Now I walk unassisted. I am free of walking aids. I keep a Canadian crutch in my car and use it when going to football and baseball games. It is useful when stepping up on curbs. I do not use the crutch when going to church, shopping, or going out to eat. I become uncomfortable standing still more than four or five minutes. This requires more strength and balance than walking.

Finger dexterity continues to challenge me. Writing, using eating utensils, turning pages in a book are routine. Picking up a coin off a counter is challenging. Being a Texas Longhorn fan, I long to give the "Hook 'em Horns" sign, holding up my index and little fingers. This I am unable to do—yet. Separation and finger dexterity are still slowly improving. I am typing these words on my computer, so my finger dexterity can't be too feeble. Neither is it very efficient.

I do not intend to give the impression this has transpired without difficulty and hard work. Following my dismissal from the rehabilitation hospital, I continued outpatient therapy three days a week for two years. While learning to use my walker, I leaned back, lost my balance and fell. My head popped back and slammed into our hardwood floor. For a few seconds I saw stars. Gratefully, my head did not dent the floor. The rule is: always lean *forward* when walking.

My second episode occurred as I stepped up on a small curb entering Luby's Cafeteria. Losing my balance I fell sideways, landing on my left arm. Hurt and embarrassed, I pondered how to get on my feet. In a few seconds two strong men were by my side hoisting me up. One inquired, "Are you hurt?"

"No, just my pride." I was mistaken. My arm continued to give me discomfort. The following day I went to my orthopedic physician to have my arm examined. An x-ray revealed my elbow was cracked. That is no big deal. In a couple of days the pain subsided, and in a matter of weeks my body repaired itself.

Other than these two episodes, I am thoroughly enjoying my retirement. There are an abundance of things to do, places to go, and friends to visit. Most important of all, I get to spend time with my wife, children, and grandchildren. This week I went to federal court and watched my son Wallace plead a case resulting in his client getting a 1.4-million-dollar judgment. Then I went to my daughter's home and spent a long time holding and loving my new great-granddaughter, Meredith. Last night Bess and I went to the Little League baseball field. We watched Lincoln, our grandson, pitch three innings. He struck out five batters. His team was leading six-to-one, when by rule a new pitcher entered the game in the fourth inning.

We recently had the joy of being present when Martha Lauren, our granddaughter, was inducted into the National Honor Society. Noble, her twin brother, who is president of the school's National Honor Socitey, presided. Later this month we will attend the high school graduation of their brother Madison. Our seven grandchildren are the joy of our lives!

Can anything be more rewarding?

Years ago I attended a retirement seminar. The speaker taught the three stages of retirement. In stage one the retiree can go anywhere. In stage two the senior citizen can go, but prefers to be closer to home and remains in the city, or state, where he resides. Travel has become more difficult. In stage three the retiree is homebound, seldom traveling out of the city.

I am still in retirement stage one, being able to go virtually anywhere. No longer do I climb mountains, wade

ving trout streams, or play golf. I am seventy-five
bably would not be doing these activities if I never
h.. BS. Growing older is a privilege not all have. I still
get up every day singing, "This is the day the Lord has
made. I will rejoice and be glad in it!" As my kids say, I am
a happy camper.

When I became ill, I lost most of my strength.
Thankfully I have never lost my sense of humor. This
happy spirit keeps my mood good and a smile on my
face. I borrowed this prayer from an unknown source.
"God grant me the senility to forget the people I never
liked anyway, the good fortune to run into the ones I do,
and the eyesight to know the difference. Amen!"

Following my dismissal from the hospital, Bess and
I have traveled extensively. We made three delightful visits to the Hawaiian Islands enjoying extended visits. Cel-
ebrating our fiftieth wedding anniversary, we took eleven
members of our family on a South Caribbean cruise.
This proved to be infinitely better than a cake-and-
punch reception. In fact, it was the best week of my life!

Beyond this we have taken cruises in the Eastern
and Western Caribbean. Our summer cruise to Alaska
defies description.

We have traveled in over twenty states since my illness. After attending my high-school fiftieth anniversary
reunion in Hot Springs, Arkansas, Bess and I drove to

246

Branson, Missouri to enjoy six outstanding shows. Departing from Branson, Bess informed me she enjoyed the shows, but does not want to ever go to Branson again. Somewhat stunned, I asked, "Why?"

"There are too many *old people* there."

"And what are we?" I asked.

"We are *not that old!*"

Texas played Michigan in the Rose Bowl January 1, 2005. We joined the Texas Exes charter flight to Los Angeles. Our accommodations were in the Century Plaza Hotel, the Texas team's hotel. Visiting with the team and coaches in the lobby was a treat. After attending the New Year's Eve dinner and party, we rose with the sun to travel with the group to the Rose Bowl Parade. Our premium seats were next to the TV cameras. Long before the parade reached where we were sitting, the sweet, fragrant scent of flowers announced the approaching floats. Following the parade we were driven to the Texas Tailgate Party featuring the Longhorn Band.

The Rose Bowl is a perfect setting for a classic football game. The Michigan and Texas University bands filled the stadium with stirring music and precision marching. The game score was so close, and exciting enough to keep the fans standing the whole game. Texas kicked a winning forty-three-yard field goal with no time remaining on the game clock.

*Wow! It doesn't get any better than that!*

A year later, January 4, 2006, Bess and I are back at the Rose Bowl watching our Texas Longhorns in the closing seconds defeat USC to win the national championship. Beyond a doubt, this is the most exciting game I have ever seen.

*It does get better!*

During April and May of 2006, we cruise the Mediterranean. After spending a few days in Lisbon we sail through the Strait of Gibraltar, stopping at Cadiz, visiting Seville, Barcelona, and Monte Carlo. We visit Livarno, taking a private tour to Pisa and Florence. Santorini is, to me, most unique and beautiful. We finish the tour visiting Malta, the ancient city of Ephesus, and finally docking at Athens.

These are not all the trips we have taken following my illness. I am not trying to share our history of travel. The point is: *There can be an active and fulfilling life after GBS.* I was a quadriplegic. My muscles had atrophied. It appeared I would never walk again. If I did manage to walk, my physical limitations would be severe. My mobility seemingly would be very limited. In reality none of these pessimistic forecasts became reality.

When we first began traveling, I would request a handicap room. I quickly discovered I did not need a handicap room. I leave the handicap room for someone who really needs it. I don't. Often handicaps are in the mind. I've given back the borrowed electric wheelchair, disposed of my regular wheelchair, donated my walker to a charitable institution, and very seldom use a cane. I am mobile, active, and happy.

My recovery and ensuing years might be titled, "Giving and Receiving." There is no joy comparable to giving. I was thrilled to give thirty-five sets of Bible commentaries to several young pastors. The bulk of my library I gave to Southwestern Baptist Theological Seminary. I gave away most of my Bibles to Austin Baptist Association. I continue the process of giving my sermons, tapes, and additional books to pastors. Bess and I have given guns, jewelry, furniture, and other personal possessions to family members and friends. What I try hard not to do is give unrequested advice.

As a senior citizen, the most precious gift I possess is time. Joyfully I spend many hours counseling churches, pastors, and laymen. I fervently hope my advice is encouraging and helpful. As often as my children and grandchildren allow, I am with them. I consider this the very best use of my time.

Pastors have a difficult time fully retiring. Consequently, I infrequently lead worship in churches. The easiest way to stay awake in church is to deliver the sermon. There is no such thing as a bad *short* sermon.

A good sermon is telling people a little less than they want to know. When I speak, I remind myself of this evident truth.

Just three years after being dismissed from the hospital, I attend the Southern Baptist Convention in Dallas and nominate Dr. Tom Elliff to be our president. Overwhelmingly he is elected. Two years later I have the honor of bringing the Convention Sermon at the Southern Baptist Convention in the Atlanta Dome. I am the first retired pastor ever given this opportunity.

While I was ill in NCC, Hyde Park Baptist Church voted to name our new planned, and now completed, family life center "The Bess and Ralph Smith Family Life Center." When the Deacons made this recommendation, they thought I was dying—or perhaps they would never have named the building in our honor. Nevertheless, Bess and I are humbly grateful for this recognition and honor.

The greatest test of character I ever faced was when I was stricken with GBS. Totally paralyzed, struggling to breathe on a respirator, months on end, I wondered If I would ever recover. If I did recuperate, would I remain a helpless quadriplegic? With superior medical help, constant encouragement from my wife, family, and friends, I did recover. Humbly, I thank every person who had such an essential part in my recovery. Without each of you I would not be writing these lines.

Most of all I thank the Great Physician, Jesus. In my darkest most depressing moments, He was always near. Life and death are ultimately in God's hands. Only by His grace do we "live and breathe and have our being."

*You Can't Fall off the Floor*

# Author's Bio

*I*n Hot Springs, Arkansas on March 19, 1931, Maggie Belle Smith had placed in her arms a ten-pound, fourteen-ounce son. She and her husband, John Morgan Smith, had waited ten months for his arrival. It did not come easy. Ralph Morgan Smith was delivered by cesarean section; his mother nearly died in the birth of her new son. His life turned out to be as unique as his birth.

After graduation from high school, Ralph moved to Fayetteville to attend the University of Arkansas. His intent was to become a lawyer, return to Hot Springs, and manage his father's businesses, which included a motel, dry-cleaning establishment, garage, service station, realty company, and liquor store. However, during his first semester in college Ralph felt called by God to be a pastor. Embarrassed by his son's life-changing decision, his father cut off all financial support.

Ralph transferred to Ouachita Baptist University to continue his college degree. With no family or financial support, this seventeen-year-old college student experienced unusual challenges. Ralph supported himself by working in construction during the summer, at the post office during Christmas, and by pastoring small country churches on the weekends.

Bess Noble Smith became Ralph's wife on June 12, 1951. He was the twenty-year-old pastor of Lake Hamilton Baptist Church. Bess had just graduated from Beaumont High School, Beaumont, Texas. They were blessed with three children: Diane, Wallace, and Peyton. Their marriage spanned fifty-six years until Bess' death following heart surgery, January 10, 2008. Dr. Smith considers his children, their spouses, and his grandchildren his greatest accomplishments in life.

Dr. Smith holds a Bachelor of Arts from Ouachita University, and a Bachelor of Divinity and a Doctor of Theology from Southwestern Baptist Theological Seminary. Additionally, Ouachita University awarded him an honorary doctorate.

Following his ministry at First Baptist Church, Rosenberg, Texas, Dr. Smith served as the senior pastor of the Hyde Park Baptist Church in Austin, Texas. Under his leadership the church became a mega-church with over 10,000 members. The church established a Child Development Center with an enrollment of 275, a school for grades K-12 with an enrollment of 850, the Hyde Park Counseling Center, and the Hyde Part Foundation. In addition, the church sponsored and started 16 churches in Austin and another in Rio De Janeiro. Brazil.

During his ministry Dr. Smith was elected president of the Baptist General Convention of Texas and president

254

of the Southern Baptist Convention Pastor's Conference. Additionally, he served as a trustee for Baylor University and as trustee chairman at Southwestern Baptist Theological Seminary. For two years he was chairman of trustees of the North American Mission Board. He is the author of six books:

*Living the Spirit-Filled Life,* published by Zondervan
*Let Me Explain,* published by Crescendo
*Facing Our Challenges with Confidence,* published by Broadman
*Helping Churches Grow,* published by Broadman
*Basic Bible Sermons on the Church,* published by Broadman

*You Can't Fall off the Floor* is the very personal story of Dr. Smith's struggle with Guillian-Barrè Syndrome, a catastrophic illness that few have been able to conquer.